MICROBLADING & NANO-BLADING COMPREHENSIVE TRAINING MANUAL

START TO FINISH
FROM NOVICE TO EXPERT

ESSENTIAL GUIDE FOR KNOWLEDGE, SKILL AND BUSINESS GROWTH

By Eveline Benjamin

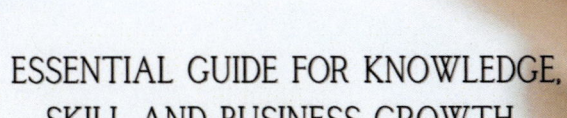

Printed in the United States of America

Published by Book Marketeers.com

"Don't be afraid, be amazing!
Success is a result of hard work, persistence, and believing in yourself!

Eveline Benjamin

Disclaimer:

This manual is designed for use as an instructor's class manual or supplementary educational material for aspiring Microblading artists. While it provides valuable information and guidance, it is essential to note that this manual alone may not be sufficient to acquire the necessary skills and practical expertise.

Proper hands-on training, as instructed in a live class environment by a qualified professional, is crucial for achieving a comprehensive understanding of the techniques outlined in this manual. The information presented here is intended to complement, not substitute, the hands-on experience and guidance provided by a skilled instructor.

Users are strongly advised to seek live training sessions under the supervision of a qualified Microblading instructor to ensure the correct application of the techniques described in this manual. Practical work experience gained in a live class setting is fundamental to mastering the art of PMU.

The author of this manual disclaims any liability or responsibility for any errors, omissions, or damages arising from the use of this material without proper hands-on training.

INTRODUCTION

Understanding Semi-Permanent Cosmetics: A Lasting Beauty Solution

Permanent cosmetics/Semi-permanent, also known as micropigmentation or cosmetic tattooing, is an innovative beauty procedure that involves depositing pigments into the skin to enhance one's facial features. This form of cosmetic enhancement offers the convenience of lasting or semi-lasting results, eliminating the need for daily makeup application. Just like any cosmetic procedures or surgeries performed to enhance the overall look of any individual, there are benefits and potential risks involved; therefore, the artist needs to fully understand and be knowledgeable about the concept of application, human skin, and client's safety.

The Process of Permanent Cosmetics:
The process of permanent cosmetics involves the use of a fine needle or a blade using a manual tool or a device to implant pigments into the skin. The procedure can be applied to various facial features, including eyebrows, eyeliner, and lip color, as well as other cosmetic enhancements like beauty marks and areola reconstruction. The pigment's color and depth are carefully chosen to achieve the desired results, and the process usually requires multiple sessions for optimal outcomes.

The Benefits of Permanent Cosmetics:
a. Time-saving and Convenience: One of the primary advantages of permanent cosmetics is the time saved in daily makeup application. This is particularly beneficial for individuals with busy

lifestyles or physical conditions that make traditional makeup application challenging.

b. Enhanced Facial Features: Permanent cosmetics can enhance and define facial features, such as fuller-looking eyebrows, more defined eyeliner, and naturally colored lips, giving a polished appearance even without traditional makeup.

c. Confidence Boost: Many individuals find that permanent cosmetics enhance their self-esteem and confidence as they wake up each day with a well-defined, aesthetically pleasing appearance.

Realistic Expectations

It's important for your clients to have realistic expectations when it comes to Microblading or Nano blading. While microblading can significantly enhance the appearance of eyebrows, it will not completely replicate the looks of a physical natural eyebrow's hair strand. The goal is to mimic natural brow hair strands by implementing pigments under the skin to create a more defined and polished look that enhances the individual's features.

Skill and Experience

The success of permanent cosmetics heavily relies on the skill and experience of the practitioner/artist. It is crucial to ensure the procedure is performed safely and accurately to achieve great healing results, happy clients and a successful business.

TABLE OF CONTENTS

Chapter 1

MICRO-BLADING

&

NANO-BLADING

We are BLADES, and we are the same technique.

MICROBLADING

Microblading is a form of tattooing; it's a technique that was originated in Asia and became popular in Europe and the U.S. around 2010. Microblading is an invasive cosmetic semi-permanent makeup procedure that is meant to last at best case scenario for 2 years' tops. The technique is performed by using a hand-held tool with a blade attached to the tip of the tool, and the reason it's called a blade is because it's made out of multiple micro-needles set in a row, creating a blade look alike. Microblades are available in many sizes, and sizes differ based on the amounts of pins and needle diameter. The main purpose of the technique is to create a natural brow look by scratching the epidermal layer of the skin, mimicking natural-looking hair strand. By doing so, brows will look fuller and better defined to frame the face. Microblading can be performed on people with existing brow hair for a fuller look or on people with no brow hair at all to create a new set of brows.

NANOBLADING

NanoBlading is the same method of application as Microblading but requires extra cautiousness due to blade size and sharpness, especially on certain skin types. The Nano blade is made out of very fine nanoneedles similar to acupuncture needles; therefore, the lines created by the blade are thinner than the Microblade. Due to blade thin size, it has the tendency to mimic vellus hair (fine hair), and as a result, it creates a much softer brow look. Important to note, it is important to explain to your clients the differences between Nano Brows (machine strokes) and Nano-Blading! When the Nano craze started a few years ago, the machine "Nano" stroke technique was referred to as Nano-blading and it created a huge confusion among clients and people who wanted to learn the technique until it was clarified to be referred to as Nano Brows or simply machine strokes technique.

To Microblade Or To Nanoblade?
(In depth in chapter 6).

Each and every blade size available on the market will offer natural-looking results; however, using the right blade based on their existing natural brow hair density will help you to achieve that natural look you seek more successfully. For example, Nano-Blade is great for women with fine brow hair like most Asian as they naturally have the fine brow hair texture or people with no brows at all, as it will provide a much softer look vs. Microblading is better for women with medium to dense hair structure like most Middle Eastern as an example.

Most women seem to suffer from partial brow loss, either due to overplucking, Thyroid problems, or generally with age as they end up slowly but surely losing the start or the ends of their brows over time. These types of brows can be tricky, especially when they have dense hair structure at the front of the brows or the middle section, missing the start of the brow or the tails and in some cases, both ends but not the middle part! Expect to have some challenging brows to work with in this field but I assure you, with every challenge comes greater knowledge as we constantly are learning from our mistakes and successes. In these cases, the combination of both Micro and Nano blades works wonders together as we are able to create strokes mimicking their existing eyebrow hair and fine hairs, creating more of a fill and a realistic look; the combination of both blades works great for women with non-existing brow hair as well.

Semi-permanent makeup is suitable for all ages with different skin types and densities but within reasons. Let's start with older skin; in most cases, they have (thin, wrinkled, dry, and some with visible large capillaries) Their skin is much easier to cut through due to being thin and that could result in pigment migration or implementing more pigment than intended if you are not cautious with your application; furthermore, most of them are already on some sort of blood thinners and medications; therefore they are prone to more than normal of pinpoint bleeding and as a result, they could heal darker in small patches in these specific spots because the old blood mixed with the pigment will inevitably heal gray/black. Some older women have tough, leathery skin surface and yet still very thin in density; I personally like to choose either nano blade or the thinnest micro blade to create my strokes on older skin; I will explain why and how in (chapter 6). It is very important and crucial to master how to control your hand pressure and the depth of your blade based on the client's skin type. I have worked on many 80+ year old women, some had a good enough skin to work with and some clients had very thin skin that I had to take extra precaution with the pressure applied. If the client has super thin skin (paper thin), they are ideally not a good candidate for the procedure. The pigment will migrate easily and they will heal ashy; you should not go through with it, and trust me, they will appreciate you once you explain your reasons and concerns to them.

The younger and healthier the skin is, the less worry we have but it's still important to determine if they are oily, normal or dry and work with each skin type as required. Nanoblading or Microblading works great for normal/Dry; their skin heals and retains the pigment better and longer. On the other hand, oily skin is prone to blurring and fading faster; it is a hit or miss with their type of skin and it is important that you are very transparent with the possible outcome and set their expectation accordingly. In my many years of experience working with oily skin, some retained the pigment and the strokes amazingly and some blurred and faded within the first 6-8 months, if not earlier; it is important to let them know that they are investing in the unknown as both you and the client cannot be sure how her skin will retain the pigment and you can give no guarantee of any kind.

A lot of women can benefit from Semi-Permanent makeup, especially women who have Alopecia, cancer patients before they start Radiotherapy/Chemotherapy, women with shaky hands or bad vision, and/or tired of having to draw their brows on every single day! However, not all women are good candidates for such invasive procedures (either for temporally reasons or permanent ones) as they might have some medical conditions of concern, like severely Diabetic people, undergoing Chemotherapy, people on Accutane, pregnant, breastfeeding and many concerning auto-immune disorders, BUT, in some cases as long as their condition is under control and they are under the supervision of a doctor, then the treating doctor can provide you with a written authorization to proceed with procedure if need be, but NEVER without a doctor's note! (In depth in chapter 3).

Eveline Benjamin

Chapter 2

SKIN FUNCTION

&

STRUCTURE

Understanding skin layers in relation to Semi-Permanent procedures

Skin biology and structure by <u>mydr</u> | <u>dermatology</u>

SKIN

The skin is the human body's largest organ, with a range of functions that support survival.

A view through the microscope reveals the layered structure of the skin and the many smaller elements within

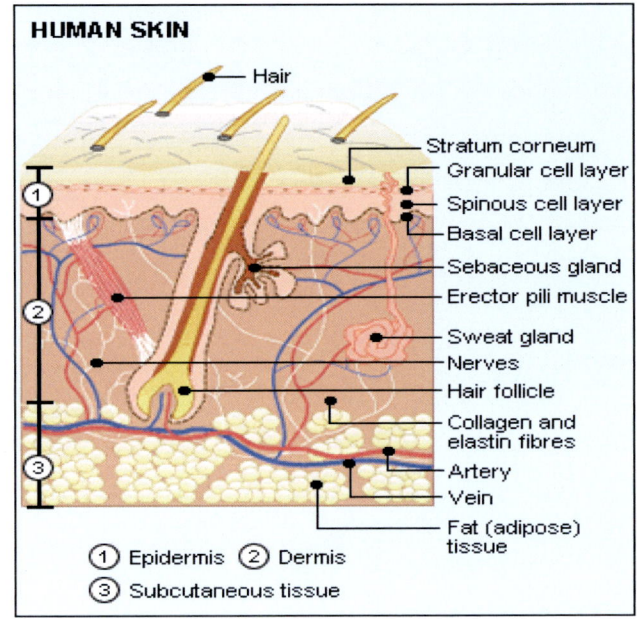

HUMAN SKIN

Hair

Stratum corneum
Granular cell layer
Spinous cell layer
Basal cell layer
Sebaceous gland
Erector pili muscle
Sweat gland
Nerves
Hair follicle
Collagen and elastin fibres
Artery
Vein
Fat (adipose) tissue

(1) Epidermis (2) Dermis
(3) Subcutaneous tissue

these layers that help the skin to perform its mainly protective role.

The skin has two main layers: the epidermis and dermis. Below these two layers is the subcutaneous ('under the skin') fat.

THE EPIDERMIS

The outer surface of the skin is the epidermis, which itself contains several layers — the basal cell layer, the spinous cell layer, the granular cell layer, and the stratum corneum. The cells in the epidermis are called keratinocytes.

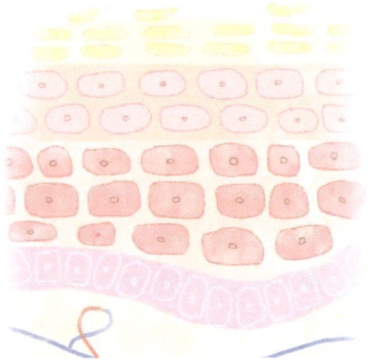

The deepest layer of the epidermis is the basal cell layer; it's where the cells are continually dividing to produce plump new skin cells (millions daily). Complete cell turnover occurs every 28 to 30 days in young adults, while the same process takes 45 to 50 days in elderly adults. These cells slowly move towards the skin surface, pushed upward by the dividing cells below them.

Blood vessels in the dermis — which is below the basal cell layer — supply nutrients to support this active growth of new skin cells. As the basal cells move upwards and away from their blood supply, their cell content and shape change.

Cells above the basal cell layer become more irregular in shape and form the spinous layer, then cells move into the granular layer, being distant from the blood supply in the dermis; the cells begin to flatten and die and accumulate a substance called keratin.

The stratum corneum ('horny layer') is the top layer of the epidermis — it is the layer of the skin that we see from the outside. Cells here are flat and scale-like in shape. These cells are dead, contain a lot of keratins and are arranged in overlapping layers that impart a tough and waterproof character to the skin's surface.

Dead skin cells continually shed from the skin's surface; this is balanced by the dividing cells in the basal cell layer to produce a state of constant renewal. Also in the basal cell layer are cells called melanocytes that produce melanin. Melanin is a pigment that is absorbed into the dividing skin cells to help protect them against damage from sunlight (ultraviolet light). The amount of melanin in your skin is determined by your genes and by how much exposure to sunlight you have. The more melanin pigment present, the darker the color of your skin.

THE DERMIS

Below the epidermis is the layer called the dermis. The top layer of the dermis — the one directly below the epidermis — has many ridges called papillae. A sample of these ridges on the fingertips, the skin's surface follows this pattern of ridges to create our individual fingerprints; however, these ridges are not on the outermost layer of skin, as it might appear.

The dermis contains a variable amount of fat, and also collagen and elastin fibers which provide strength and flexibility to the skin. In an <u>older person,</u> the elastin fibers fragment and much of the skin's elastic quality is lost, along with the loss of subcutaneous fat, resulting in wrinkles. When the skin is exposed to sunlight, modified cholesterol in the dermis produces vitamin D, which helps the body to absorb calcium for healthy bones.

<u>Here are some of the other structures within the dermis that enhance the skin's function</u>

- Blood vessels supply nutrients to the dividing cells in the basal layer and remove any waste products. They also help maintain body temperature by dilating and carrying more blood when the body needs to lose heat from its surface; they narrow and carry less blood when the body needs to limit the amount of heat lost at its surface.

- Specialized nerves in the dermis detect heat, cold, pain, pressure and touch and relay this information to the brain. In this way, the body senses changes in the environment that may potentially harm the body.

- Hair follicles are embedded in the dermis and occur all over the body, except on the soles, palms and lips. Each hair follicle has a layer of cells at its base that continually divides, pushing overlying cells upwards inside the follicle. These cells become keratinized and die, like the cells in the epidermis, but here forms the hair shaft that is visible above the skin. The color of the hair is determined by the amount and type of melanin in the outer layer of the hair shaft.

- A sebaceous ('oil') gland opens into each hair follicle and produces sebum, a lubricant for the hair and skin that helps repel water, damaging chemicals and microorganisms ('germs').

- Attached to each hair follicle are small erector pili muscle fibers. These muscle fibers contract in cold weather and sometimes in fright — this pulls the hair up which pulls on the skin with the result being 'goosebumps.

- Sweat glands occur on all skin areas — each person has more than 2 million. When the body needs to lose heat, these glands produce sweat (a mix of water, salts and some waste material). Sweat moves to the skin's surface via the sweat duct, and evaporation of this water from the skin has a cooling effect on the body.

The skin varies in thickness and the number of hair follicles, sebaceous glands and sweat glands in different areas of the body. The thickest skin is on the soles of the feet and the palms of the hands and the largest number of hair follicles are on the top of the head.

SUBCUTANEOUS FAT

The innermost layer of the skin is the layer of subcutaneous fat, and its thickness varies in different regions of the body. The fat stored in this layer represents an energy source for the body and helps to insulate the body against changes in the outside temperature.

FUNCTIONS OF THE SKIN

As you can see, there are many different structures within the skin. Together, these structures impart many protective properties to the skin that help avoid damage to the body from outside influences. In this way, the skin:

- Protects the body from water loss and any form of injury due to bumps, chemicals, sunlight, or microorganisms.

- Helps to control body temperature;

- Is a sensor to inform the brain of changes in the immediate environment.

- Synthesizes vitamin D.

THE EPIDERMIS & MICROPIGMENTATION

Now that we learned about the Epidermal layer of the skin, we have a better understanding why Microblading and Nanoblading are referred to as Semi-Permanent; with every cell turnover, we are constantly shedding dead skin and along with it, the implanted pigment, through the continuation of this normal skin function the pigment will slowly fade and completely be gone if the client chooses not to continue getting the procedure. It is another reason why these procedures have gained popularity over the years, unlike the traditional permanent makeup where the pigments are implanted in the actual Dermis and it can last for almost 20+. Another benefit of implanting the pigment in the Epidermis is that we are able to create the strokes without the risk of any pigment migration in the skin since the depth of the blade is superficial; furthermore, the pigment will not change color over time like traditional permanent makeup since it sheds off with the skin unless of course we choose unreliable cheap pigments or if the client is careless in protecting the implanted pigment from external factors and the environment.

The average thickness of forehead skin is 1.70 mm; however, the Epidermis varies in thickness from one person to another, but on average, it's thicker or thinner from what is shown in the photo below.

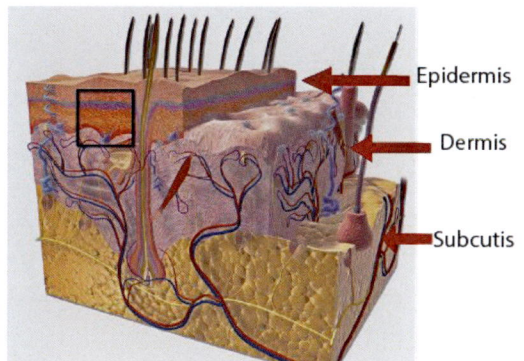

Epidermis

Dermis

Subcutis

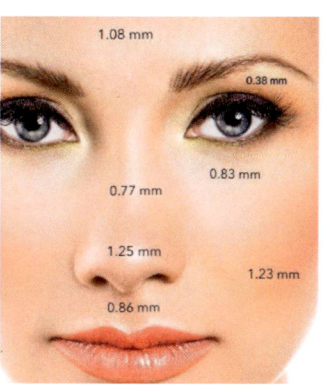

Eveline Benjamin

Chapter 3

CONTRAINDICATIONS

CONTRAINDICATION

There are many Health and skin issues (temporary issues or permanent ones) that can prevent the client from getting any form of tattooing done. Not all, but in some cases, if the client desires to proceed with getting the procedure, their Medical Provider or Dermatologist should authorize the PMU procedure and email the authorization directly to you. The risk of working on such skin will lead to excessive bleeding, infection, undesired discoloration of pigment and a high risk for worse flare-ups of their condition. Taking your extreme precautions is very important for the sake of your client as well as yourself. Here are some of the most common contraindications that you might come across.

PSORIASIS

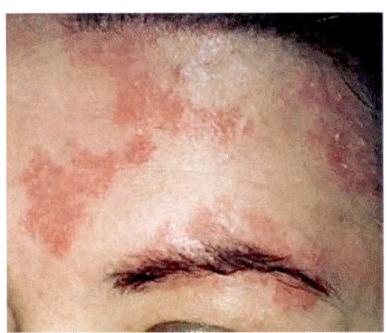

Psoriasis is an auto-immune system disorder where infection-fighting cells attack healthy skin cells by mistake, causing patches of thick red skin and silvery scales. Patches are typically found on the elbows, knees, scalp, lower back, face, palms, and soles of feet but can affect other places. Triggers include infections, stress, and cold. If the client has a history of Psoriasis on their face, it is best to avoid the procedure because it can trigger a flair-up, but if the client doesn't normally get these patches around their brow area and still want to go through with the procedure, have her sign a waiver and request a dermatologist approval letter to be emailed to you directly.

DERMATITIS

Dermatitis is a general term for conditions that cause inflammation of the skin. Examples include atopic dermatitis (eczema), contact dermatitis, and seborrheic dermatitis (dandruff). These conditions cause red rashes, dry skin, and itchiness among other symptoms. Dermatitis can be managed by a healthcare provider or a dermatologist.

Contact dermatitis:

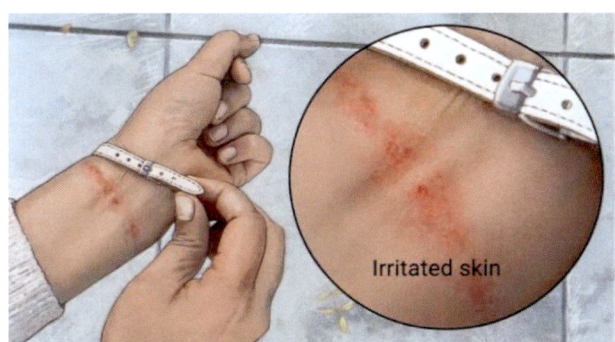

A skin rash caused by contact with a certain substance. The substance might irritate the skin or trigger an allergic reaction. Some common substances include soap, cosmetics, fragrances, jewelry, and poison ivy. The main symptom is a red rash wherever the skin comes into contact with the irritant. Avoiding the irritant or allergen should allow the rash to clear in two to four weeks. Creams or medications can help reduce itching. The rash isn't contagious and the procedure can be performed after being treated and cleared 100%.

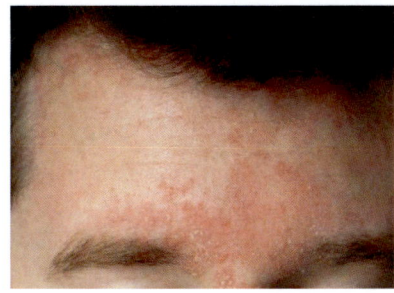

source "*Photo by Healthjade.net*"

Seborrheic dermatitis on the face:

Seborrheic dermatitis causes a rash of oily patches with yellow or white scales. The rash may look darker or lighter in people with brown or black skin and redder in those with white skin. It is a noncontagious skin condition. Not a candidate and must not go through with the procedure because the condition will worsen and pigment will never retain due to the inflammation and the amount of oil in the skin.

Atopic dermatitis:

Photo by Dermatology center of Indiana

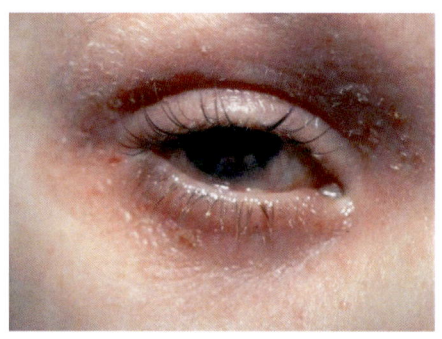

(Eczema) is a condition that causes dry, itchy and inflamed skin; the symptoms can appear anywhere on the body and vary widely from person to person. Atopic dermatitis is long lasting (chronic) and tends to flare sometimes. It can be irritating but it's not contagious. If the client has a history of eczema on their face, it is best to avoid the procedure because it can trigger a flair-up, but if the client doesn't normally get this inflammation around their brow area and still wants to go through with the procedure, have her sign a waiver and request a dermatologist approval letter to be emailed directly to you.

KELOID

"All wounds heal through scar formation. There are different types of scars: atrophic scars, hypertrophic scars, and keloids. Usually, scars are hyperpigmented and raised for a couple of months. It will then mature and look better after a year or two. For those who are keloid formers, their scars continue to grow bigger than the original wound indefinitely.

Can microblading cause scars and keloids? Microblading, if done too deep or if it gets infected, may lead to scars or hypertrophic scars. However, keloid formation or thick, enlarged and elevated scars on the face are rare.

Keloid scar formation

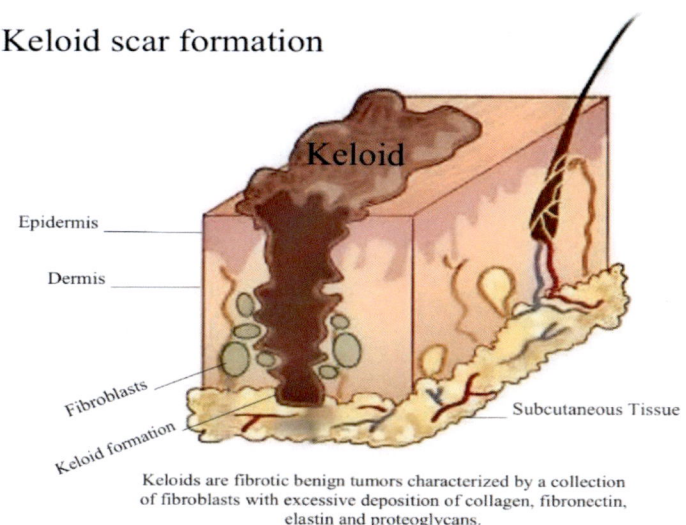

Keloids are fibrotic benign tumors characterized by a collection of fibroblasts with excessive deposition of collagen, fibronectin, elastin and proteoglycans.

If you are prone to hypertrophic scars or keloids, you can still do eyebrow microblading but choose wisely who will do the procedure.

Unlike ordinary makeup, microblading or permanent makeup involves cutting or poking the skin to implant the ink. Cutting the skin at the correct level needs a lot of practice and skill before one can master microblading. Best to trust and choose those who have been doing the procedure for years now."

Article (September 2, 2021) ...written by Dr. Aicee Bernal, a Plastic and Reconstructive Surgeon and Permanent Makeup Artist based in Manila, Philippines, since 2013

Personally, I would not recommend machine strokes as this technique can most likely lead to deeper needle penetration in the skin and trigger keloid. However, blading can be done indeed **only** if you know the skin well and you have mastered your technique and more so can control the depth of the blade with extreme precautions. **Master your skills and blade depth first and <u>until then</u> please do NOT attempt to work on people who are prone to Keloid.**

MOLES & BIRTHMARKS

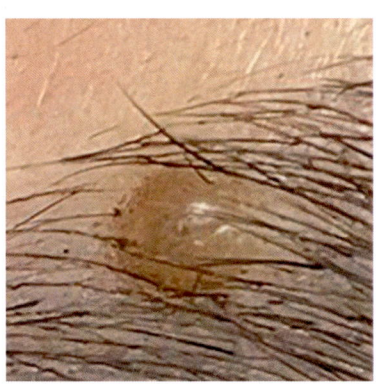

<u>A mole</u> is made of many cells clustered together instead of being distributed evenly; some people happen to have a mole or two located in the brow area or close to the hairline; it is unfortunate to the client as the mole cannot be worked on with a blade, it will never retain the pigment not to mention risking the fact that it can be cancerous (although rare but can develop into melanoma), therefore, it should be completely avoided during pigment application and the artist must work around it. In some cases, the client has existing hair to cover the mole which helps the overall look after the procedure, but for those who don't, they need to be informed ahead of time of what to expect before starting the procedure.

<u>Birthmarks</u>:

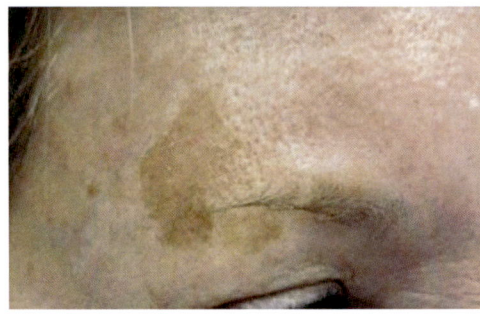

Birthmarks are common in many people; it presents itself on the skin at birth or soon after. Birthmarks can be flat or raised and, in most cases, they are benign; however, sometimes they can be linked to some diseases or even cancer, therefore, avoiding the mark altogether is important to avoid problems. Some clients may seek medical laser treatment to remove the birthmark; if so, it must be fully healed before performing Microblading or the Nanoblading procedure.

LESIONS

Any open lesions, rashes, blisters should not be worked on until they are fully healed; the risk of infection and skin damage would be inevitable in these cases.

ROSACEA | ACNE ROSACEA

Rosacea is a common chronic but treatable skin condition effecting mainly the face but can be seen on the neck and the chest as well. People with Rosacea condition suffer from long- 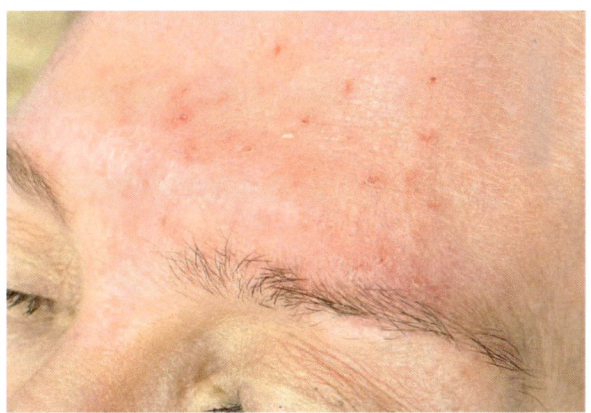 term redness, burning and stinging sensations with visible small blood vessel bumps that can be pustules as well (Acne Rosacea). People with acne Rosacea on the brows or borderline should not undergo PMU brow procedures unless the condition is totally under control with medication and a clearance from a dermatologist has been emailed to you.

ALLERGIES

In regards to allergies, as we know it all varies from one person to another as well as the severity. Some people, they know exactly what they are allergic to and some say they were never tested and can never tell what causes certain rashes or hives on their skin. It is always best to do an allergy patch test with a nude color pigment behind the ear and allow 24-72 hours for any reaction on the skin to form. If all is clear then there is nothing to worry about. I also advice to always use Nitrile gloves and latex-free Gauzes. People can have allergies to: -

- Latex

- Colors

- Metals, including but not limited to stainless steel and nickel, (Iron oxide contains nickel) found in pigments and can be found in brow pencils and makeup.

- Numbing agents like Lidocaine, Tetracaine, Benzocaine, Epinephrine, and Prilocaine.

ACCUTANE

Isotretinoin (Accutane) is an oral drug used to treat severe acne. While taking isotretinoin, the skin may be more sensitive to the sun, fragile, risk of scarring, and prone to skin infections. Cosmetic procedures, such as hair removal methods like waxing, dermabrasion, laser treatments, and PMU procedures should be delayed until the client has been off isotretinoin for at least 6-12 months or as directed by their doctor. Isotretinoin is available in a variety of brand names, including Absorica, Amnesteem, Claravis, Myorisan, and Sotret. The original brand, *Accutane*, is no longer on the market; however, the drug is sometimes still referred to by this name. "Can Accutane use cause skin thinning? There is no scientific link confirming that Accutane use results in skin thinning. *Says Valerie Hanft, MD, Board Certified Dermatologist*".

STEROIDS

Corticosteroid medicines (cortisone, hydrocortisone and prednisone) are medicines used to treat rheumatoid arthritis, inflammatory bowel disease, asthma, allergies and many other conditions. While on these medications, the epidermis starts thinning and changes the structural layer in the dermis especially when it is given in a topical form. When this happens, the skin can become lax, wrinkled, shiny, thin, bruises as well as the tendency of slower wound healing. Due to these factors, any cosmetics procedure, including PMU procedures must wait for 6 months after stopping the treatment or as permitted by their doctor.

THYROID

Thyroid disease is very common, with an estimated 20 million people in the Unites States having some type of thyroid disorder. A woman is about five to eight times more likely to be diagnosed with a thyroid condition than a man. A person could either have Hyperthyroidism or Hypothyroidism which can be confirmed with blood test. The disease can be hereditary, linked to medical conditions like Type 1 diabetes, autoimmune disorders and other conditions and/or by taking medication that's high in iodine. Types of thyroid disorders associated with hyper- or hypothyroidism:

- Thyroiditis.
- Graves' disease.
- Hashimoto's disease.
- Goiter.
- Thyroid nodule.
- Thyroid cancer.

Although it is safe to work on people with Thyroid disease, PMU results cannot be guaranteed nor predicted and that is due to hormones fluctuation and thyroid functions. Their skin might not retain the pigment well and the overall healing results as well as the healed color cannot be predicted. It is always wise to inform clients of this possibility during the consultation to make them well aware before investing.

LUPUS

Lupus is a disease that occurs when your body's immune system attacks your own tissues and organs (autoimmune disease). Inflammation caused by lupus can affect many different body systems — including your joints, skin, kidneys, blood cells, brain, heart, and lungs. PMU on People with lupus should be taken with a high level of seriousness because they are more vulnerable to infection as both the disease and its treatments can weaken the immune system; their healing process is slow, not to mention the possibility of triggering a flare-up of the condition. It is very important to get their doctor's clearance in order to attempt working on their skin.

With that being said, since PMU is a form of tattooing, a 2019 study on tattoos in people with lupus can ease your mind a little but does not mean we should never take the precautions needed for the sake of our client's health.

Lupus. September 28, 2019 PupMed https://pubmed.ncbi.nlm.nih.gov/31382852/

Objective: The objective of this study was to determine the safety of tattoos in patients with systemic lupus erythematosus (SLE).

Methods: Patients (N = 147; ≤55 years; 92% women) were asked if they had tattoos. The characteristics of the tattoos and the immediate complications were investigated and compared with those of a matched control group. We examined retrospectively after the tattoo was completed whether there had been flare-ups or increased organ damage (Systemic Lupus International Collaborating Clinics/American College of Rheumatology Damage Index (SDI)). Finally, we compared the SLE-related characteristics of patients with and without tattoos.

Results: Twenty-eight patients (19%, 26 women, median (interquartile range) age 33 (25-42) years, 65 tattoos in total) had ≥1 tattoo. At the time the tattoo was done, the median (interquartile range) SLEDAI and SDI were 2 (0-2) and 0 (0-1), respectively. The characteristics of the tattoos were similar to those of controls. No patients experienced acute complications. After a median follow-up of 17 (12-20) months (3 (2-4) visits/year) four patients had five mild-to-moderate flare-ups. The median time between the tattoo and the flare-up was 9 (6-14) months. No increase in SDI was observed. The SLE-related characteristics of patients with and without tattoos were similar.

✓ **Conclusion:** Tattoos seem to be safe in SLE patients with **inactive or low active disease.**

In general, can Autoimmune disease patients get Micropigmentation?

In full honesty, there are many autoimmune diseases that can be listed; some are more serious than others; it is best to take your precautions and use your best judgment in this case. Whichever PMU technique is used, whether machine or blades, we are cutting into the skin, and for the individuals with **active or untreated autoimmune diseases,** it is best not to work with these conditions for the safety of our client's sake, these conditions can severely impact the healing process of the individuals and their health. A doctor's clearance letter or email is a must in order for the procedure to take place even when the disease is not active; that way, you are watching out for your client as well as yourself. For example, you can proceed with the procedure on some mild cases like a thyroid patient that their condition is supervised and controlled with medication through their doctor without a doctor's note, but if their thyroid is cancerous then their doctor must be informed and an email clearance from the doctor must be obtained before scheduling the procedure.

DIABETES

Diabetes is a chronic (long-lasting) health condition that affects how your body turns food into energy. With diabetes, your body doesn't make enough insulin or can't use it as well as it should. When there isn't enough insulin or cells stop responding to insulin, too much blood sugar stays in your bloodstream. Over time, that can cause serious health problems, such as heart disease, vision loss, and kidney disease and delayed healing from injuries or wounds. There are a few types of diabetes, and a doctor's clearance is important, especially type 1 diabetes. (Some cases are so severe, best not to perform the procedure on them)

"In short, having diabetes per se does not mean you can't have microblading done. You just need to take medications that will regulate your blood sugar levels before doing the procedure".

Dr. Aicee Bernal, a board-certified plastic and reconstructive surgeon and permanent makeup expert.

CHEMOTHERAPY/ RADIATION

Certain cancer treatments (such as chemotherapy, radiation therapy, surgery, stem cell or bone marrow transplant, or steroids) and the cancer itself can suppress or weaken the immune system. These treatments can lower the number of white blood cells and other immune system cells, leaving cancer patients prone to infections very easily.

Their skin is also compromised due to the treatments, therefore if the client wishes to get a PMU procedure done, the client would need to get it done before starting the treatments or after but never during. A period of 8 weeks after finishing the treatment is what is recommended for the client to wait before getting their brows done, and the client's oncologist's approval is needed first along with a letter from the office or an email directed to you before proceeding.

PREGNANT/ NURSING

Working on a pregnant woman or while nursing should be denied by the technician. There are no studies on the possible negative effects or risks that can affect the fetus/baby; for that reason alone any PMU procedures should never be performed on a pregnant woman or a nursing mother. Furthermore, an average of 3–6-month period after stopping breastfeeding is required because unbalanced hormones play a big factor in the final healed PMU results as well as the retention. Pregnant women are prone to skin changes during pregnancy, changes like becoming oily, dry and in most cases, develop melasma. Also, numbing agent can be a problem as well, especially the ones containing epinephrine, as it may be linked to fetal cardiac problems.

HIV / HEPATITIS

It is best not to work on individuals with transmittable blood diseases such as HIV or Hepatitis as these conditions tremendously impact the individual's immune system and healing process. For these reasons and for the safety of the individuals as well as yours, it is best to refrain from performing the procedure. Also, please keep in mind, not every individual out there is aware that they carry the disease, so please make sure to always follow the rules of sanitation and sterilization and treat every client as they can be with blood-borne pathogens to eliminate the risk or cross contamination.

Chapter 4

FITZPATRICK

&

SKIN UNDERTONES

FITZPATRICK SCALE

Developed by Dr. Thomas Fitzpatrick and it is originally used to measure the skin type's ability to tolerate sun exposure. It is also used as a helpful tool in micro-pigmentation since the pigment implanted in the skin interacts directly with the melanin, determining the final result of the healed color. According to this scale, skin types are classified from 1 to 6 and take into account the characteristics of hair color, skin color, and eye color. These structures are used because they have a particular component in common, melanin. Pigmentation of the skin results from the accumulation of melanin created by the melanocytes in the epidermis. Differences in skin pigmentation result both from the relative ratio of eumelanin (brown–black), responsible for the darkness of the human skin, and pheomelanin (yellow–red) which is responsible for the skin undertone, as well as the number of melanosomes (membrane-bound) within melanocytes. The overall melanin density correlates with the darkness of the skin as well as Fitzpatrick skin type.

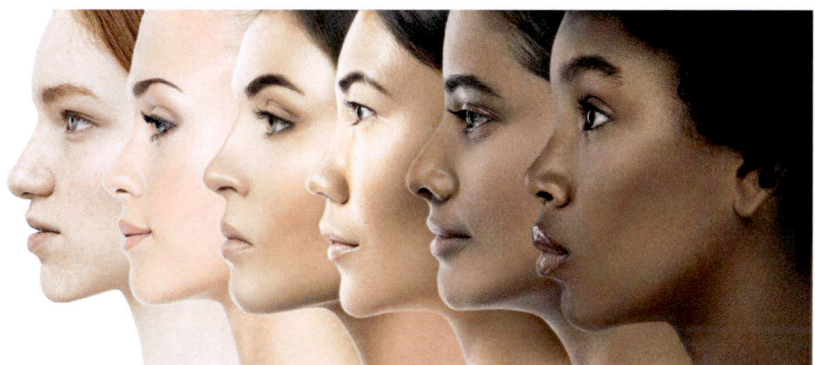

Skin Type 1	Skin Type 2	Skin Type 3	Skin Type 4	Skin Type 5	Skin Type 6
Pale white skin/ red or blonde hair, blue or green eyes, freckles	White, fair skin/ blonde or light hair/ blue, green or hazel eyes	Creamy white skin/ light to dark hair/ light or dark eye color	Olive skin/ brown hair/ brown eyes	Dark skin/ dark hair/ brown or black eyes	Very dark or black skin/ dark brown or black hair/ brown or black eyes
Always burns, never tans	Usually burns, tans with difficulty	Burns mildly, tans gradually	Rarely burns, tans with ease	Very rarely burns, tans very easily	Never burns, tans very easily

Fitzpatrick Scale Questioner

Score	Analysis	0	1	2	3	4
	What is the color of your eyes?	Light Blue, or light Green	Grey, Green or Hazel	Blue	Brown	Brownish Black
	What is the natural color of your hair?	Sandy Red	Blonde	Chestnut, Sark blonde	Dark Brown	Black
	What is the color of your skin? (Unexposed areas)	Reddish	Very Fair	Fair with Beige or Olive tint	Light Brown, Olive	Dark Brown
	Do you have freckles/sun spots on sun-exposed areas?	Many	several	Few	Incidental	None
	What happens when you stay in the sun too long?	Painful redness, blistering, peeling	Blistering followed by peeling	Burns, sometimes followed by peeling	Rarely burns	Never had burns
	To what degree do you turn Brown?	Hardly or not at all	Light color tan	Reasonable tan	Tan very easily	Turn dark Brown quickly
	Do you turn brown several hours after sun exposure?	Never	Seldom	Sometimes	Often	Always
	How does your face respond to the sun?	Very sensitive	Sensitive	Normal	Very resistant	Never had a problem
	When did you last expose yourself to the sun, tanning bed, or self-tanning creams?	More than 3 months ago	2-3 month ago	1-2 month ago	Less than 1 month ago	Less than 2 weeks ago
	Do you expose the area to be treated to the sun?	Never	Hardly ever	Sometimes	Often	Always

Total	Score	Fitzpatrick Skin Type
	0-7	I
	8-16	II
	17-25	III
	25-30	IV
	Over 30	V - VI

Although, Fitzpatrick scale is great to determine our clients' skin types, we definitely need to keep in mind that in this day and age, we are dealing with multi-racial and mixed ethnicities which sometimes can make it a little more confusing to pin point the type 100%. Also, people nowadays are big fans of tanning which is another factor that make it hard to determine their natural skin tones just from the looks of their skin; that's why it is best to always ask the basic questions or better have your client fill out Fitzpatrick scale questioner to better determine their true skin type. There are also some Electronic Fitzpatrick Skin Tone Analyzer on the market that can be a helpful digital tool as well.

SKIN UNDERTONE

Skin undertone isn't the same thing as your natural tone or the color of your naked skin; it refers to the subtle hues beneath the surface of the skin. Now that we know that our body creates two different types of melanin pigments (Eumelanin and Pheomelanin) in the melanocyte that bring forth our human skin color, let us focus on the three traditional undertones: **warm, cool, and neutral** and all three are determined by the amount of Pheomelanin melanin (yellow-red) levels and their distribution in the skin.

- Warm Undertone: Their skin is a yellow, peachy, or golden hue. Warm undertones are commonly associated with individuals who have darker skin tones but can also be found in people with lighter skin. Some characteristics of warm undertones include a tendency to tan easily and veins that appear more greenish.

- Cool Undertones: Their skin is pink, rosy, or bluish hue. Cool undertones are frequently found in individuals with fair or light skin, but they can also be present in people with medium to dark skin. Those with cool undertones may be more prone to sunburn and often have veins that appear purple/blue.

- Neutral Undertones: They are a blend of warm and cool undertones. Individuals with neutral undertones typically have a good balanced melanin levels in their skin, so they are neither cool or warm and their veins may appear to be a mix of green, purple and blue.

When you implant the pigment in the skin, it interacts with the level of melanin to get the final color, which is a reason why the same pigment used sets differently per the individual; therefore, it is important to be familiar with Fitzpatrick scale and how to determine skin undertone as well as being familiar with the pigment base color of the brand you will be using, altogether will determine the perfect color for your client. It can be somewhat challenging at first but I promise you it gets easier with time. Here are my 3 favorite methods that I personally trust to determine the skin undertone and help choose the right pigment base.

- Check out your veins. One of the easiest ways to predict undertones is through visible veins on the skin. For example, if the veins look greenish, then the person has yellow/warm undertones. People with purplish-looking veins are red/cool undertones and if the person has neutral undertones, you see a mixture of both warm and cool tones (purple, green, blue); keep in mind, some people have thicker skin than others which makes it harder to see their veins, so you would need to use some of the other methods to determine the undertone.

- Are nail beds pink or peach? If nail beds are yellow/peachy color then the undertone is warm; if they are pinkish then the undertone is cool; and if neither then they are neutral.

- Do they look best in gold or silver jewelry? If their answer is sliver then they are cool undertone; if they answer gold then they are warm undertone; and if they believe they look good with both then they are neutral.

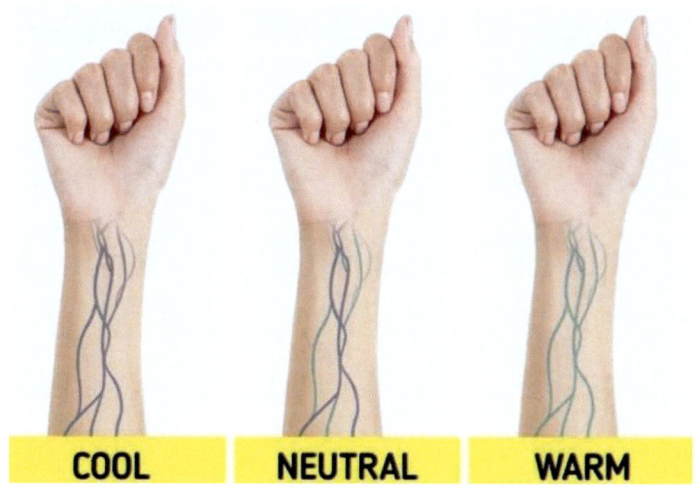

Credit: @eklescare via Instagram

Eveline Benjamin

Chapter 5

COLOR THEORY

WHAT IS COLOR THEORY

Color theory is a field of study that explores how colors interact, how they can be combined, and how they affect human perception and emotions; it is essential in various fields, including art, design, psychology, and even marketing. Here are some key aspects of color theory:

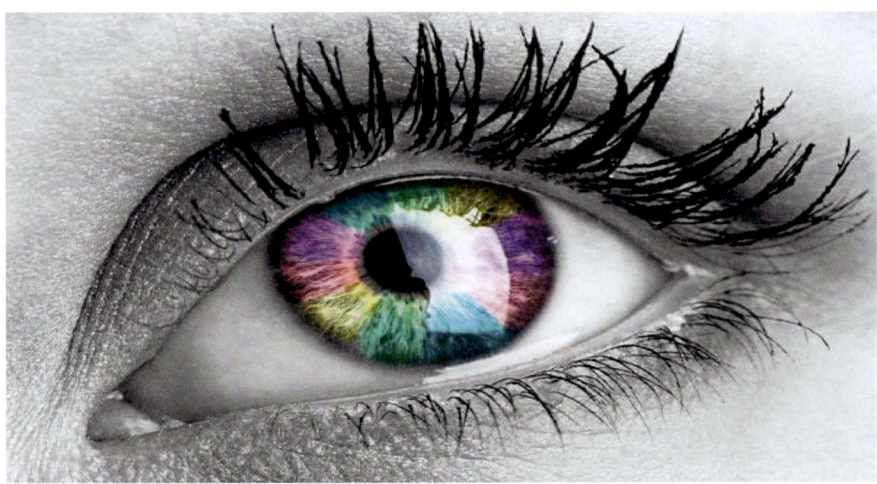

UNDERSTANDING COLOR

There are three main classifications to colors: primary, secondary, and tertiary colors.

Thereafter, classifications become more complex depending on the combinations of colors between and among the main classifications.

Primary colors: Red, blue and yellow. These are the basic colors that cannot be created by mixing other colors yet they represent the base colors that all other colors originate from.

Secondary colors: These colors are created by mixing two primary colors together. Green (blue + yellow), Orange (red + yellow), and purple/violet (red + blue).

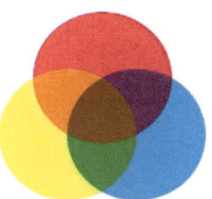

Tertiary colors: They are colors made by mixing a primary color with a secondary color. Examples (reddish orange) (yellowish green) etc.

COLOR PROPERTIES

Colors can be described in terms of having three main characteristics:

Hue: Refers to the specific color itself, such as red, blue, or green. It is what we typically think of when we refer to a color.

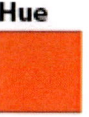

Hue

Saturation: Also known as chroma or intensity, refers to the purity or vividness of a color. Highly saturated colors are vibrant, while desaturated colors appear more muted.

Saturation

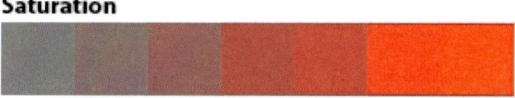

Brightness: Also called value, refers to how light or dark a color appears. (Adding black makes the color darker and white makes the color lighter).

Brightness

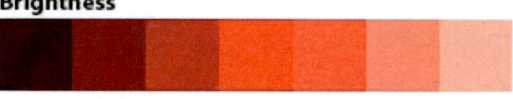

Colors are classified as cool, warm, and neutral colors.

WARM COLORS are made of RED, ORANGE, and YELLOW.

COOL COLORS are made of GREEN, BLUE, and PURPLE/VIOLET.

NEUTRAL COLORS or earth tones are black, gray, brown, beige, tan, and white.

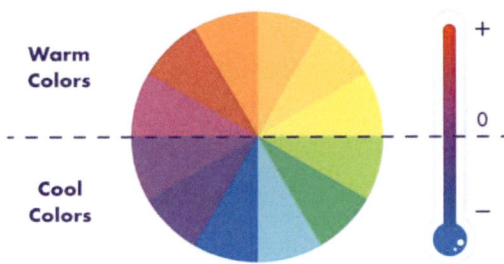

UNDERSTANDING COMPLEMENTARY COLORS:

They are two colors that are opposite of each other on the color wheel. They enhance each other and when combined or mixed, they cancel each other out.

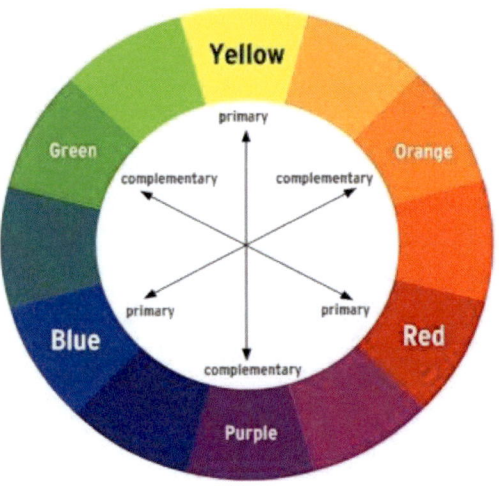

The complementary colors are one secondary color and the primary color that is not contained in that secondary color.

For example, purple contains blue and red and is, therefore, a secondary color. Its complementary color is yellow. Applying yellow over the purple will cause both colors to mute and look nothing like how they originated.

The complementary colors are:

1. Purple and yellow

2. Orange and blue

3. Green and yellow

Complementary colors are used often for color correction on brows; when mixed, they cancel each other out.

Brown is a neutral color and is widely used in PMU applications

It can be created by mixing the three primary colors together or by mixing the complementary colors together.

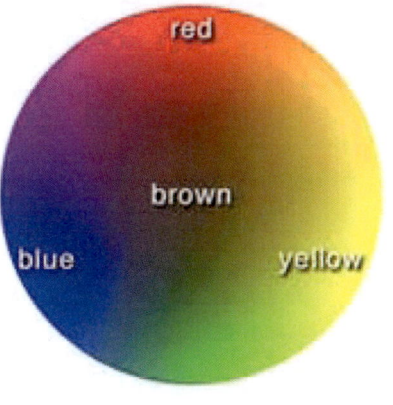

Brown color temperature can be due to:

- When the primary color of the base is blue or green, then it is a cool brown.

- When the primary color of the base is red or orange, then it is a warm brown.

- When the primary color of the base is purple (red and blue) the brown is neutral.

Color theory plays a crucial role in the realm of permanent makeup. A thorough understanding of the color wheel, undertones, skin tones, and pigment selection enables artists to create harmonious and realistic enhancements. Skillful application, combined with an awareness of the healing process and pigment fading, ensures that clients can enjoy long-lasting and visually pleasing results from their permanent makeup procedures. As the field of permanent makeup continues to evolve, artists must remain knowledgeable and adaptable to meet the diverse needs of their clientele.

Color Wheel in Permanent Makeup & Color correction: The color wheel is a valuable tool for permanent makeup artists to choose the right modifier pigments. Complementary colors are opposite each other on the color wheel and as I mentioned above when combined, two complementary colors will dull and neutralize/cancel each other out, resulting in a neutral color. This is because combining two complementary colors is the same as mixing all three primary colors. **An example of complementary colors is green and red; when mixed, green + red = neutral brown, using orange (warm) corrector or modifier will neutralize a blue/grey eyebrow back to a neutral brown, same as using green will neutralize red/orang eyebrow back to brown**. Understanding complementary colors can help you to choose a suitable color during the touch-up or color corrections.

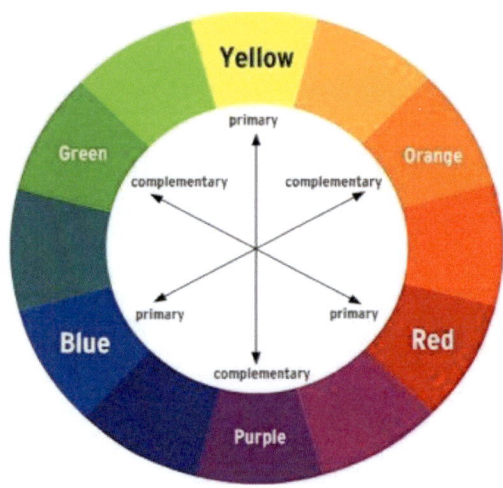

Chapter 6

PMU PIGMENTS

Organic. In-Organic . Hybrid . Allergies & MSDS

PIGMENTS

What is the difference between tattoo ink and pigment?

Permanent makeup tattoo pigments are diluted; therefore, this allows for a more natural and softer color in the skin vs. traditional tattoo inks that are much more concentrated, which means that they are much stronger in color and vivid. Although permanent makeup pigments are in liquid form, just like tattoo ink, the retention in the skin is different due to the depth of application and color concentration. Permanent makeup pigments are implemented in the upper layer of the skin and will stay in the skin for months before the body starts to slowly break it down, not to mention the natural cell turnover of shedding the pigment along with the dead skin, resulting in a complete fading of the pigment, which is great for the client who wishes to not continue with the annual application. Tattoo ink implantation in the skin is much deeper, resulting in permanent retention and the body breaks it down in a much slower pace and not nearly enough to fade the ink.

When performing a PMU procedure, you want to use the best pigments for your clients; you also want to be aware of their base color tone and the origin. Pigments are classified into 3 groups: **organic**, **inorganic**, and in the recent year's **hybrid** (A formula made up of mixing both organic and inorganic pigments). Most PMU pigments available on the market now contain both organic and inorganic elements to them which makes it the perfect combination to get the best of both for best-healed results.

ORGANIC VS. INORGANIC PIGMENTS

Organic Pigments

Organic pigments are carbon-based compounds. Pigments that were animal and plant derivatives weren't the best option as the animals and plants particles would often cause allergic reactions. These pigments now are synthetic, meaning they are human-made and mostly made from hydrogen and carbon from lakes and dyes. The synthesis of organic pigments allows for precise control over color, stability, and safety. These pigments are extensively tested for the use in cosmetics to ensure they meet strict quality and safety standards before being used in permanent makeup procedures.

Pros of Organic Pigments

- Organic pigments consist usually of smaller particles and are more transparent.

- Organic pigments tend to be more vibrant and have a wider range of colors.

- Organic particles are bright, quick to implant, and long-lasting.

- Organic pigments are often considered better for oily skin. Due to the finer particle size that allows the pigment to integrate more evenly into the skin, making it less susceptible to migration and fading.

Cons of Organic Pigments

Because of the small particles of carbon found in organic pigments, the retention is much longer than inorganic pigments, causing slow fading which is good in a lot of cases but because its slow fading, it will eventually fade into a cooler color (Ashy/gray).

Inorganic Pigments

Inorganic pigments are made by adding iron oxide elements to other substances. They are derived from natural dry ground minerals and they are called "inorganic" pigments because they're made from synthetic metals such as manganese, titanium oxide, and ultramarines. The particles inside inorganic pigments are much larger than organic pigments and therefore have more coverage. Just like organic pigments, they are now solely produced in a lab.

Pros of Inorganic Pigments

- Inorganic pigments are beautiful, muted, earthy tones and are very stable in color.

- Inorganic consists of larger particles which means more passes are required to get the desired saturation, promote gradual saturation of pigment.

- Inorganic pigments fade faster.

- Inorganic pigments can also withstand the sun and are opaque.

Cons of Inorganic Pigments

Inorganic pigments fade faster and would require frequent touch-ups; they also fade into warm tones such as orange or reddish; these are easy fixes, much easier to fix than organic pigments.

Organic VS Inorganic Pigments	
Organic	**Inorganic**
Carbon based	Natural Mineral based
Particle size: Small	Particle size: Large
Intensity: Bright & Vivid	Intensity: Soft & Earthy
Saturation: Fast	Saturation: Slower
Opacity: Low – Translucent	Opacity: High - Opaque
Slow Fading	Faster Fading
Usually Ash/Gray fading	Usually Warm/Red fading

HYBRID PIGMENTS

Hybrid pigment formulations have a blend of both organic and inorganic pigment particles and they are becoming very popular. By combining both pigment types, we are able to take the benefits of each - for optimized color brightness, opacity, and ideal longevity. However, not all hybrid pigments are created equally. There is a whole spectrum of hybrid pigments. Some may be organic-based and some are inorganic-based. This line of pigment is fairly new and seems promising for better-healed results.

WHEN TO USE ORGANIC-BASED PIGMENT OR INORGANIC-BASED PIGMENTS?

Now that we have learned about the different types of pigments, we come to ask when to use one or the other? It is pretty simple when you put in consideration of the skin type you are working with, including the client's undertone, skin density, and the client's expectations and desired result.

Inorganic pigments are less permanent compared to organic, providing flexibility for clients who do not wish to commit permanently to a specific shape or color; they also offer the opportunity for frequent touch-ups due to the faster fading than the organic pigment, allowing needed adjustment to the shape and color for your clients as they age. These pigments are preferred to be used on thin or mature skin, clients with fair skin and sun-damaged skin, also for those clients that have the tendency to pull cool or dark. It is also a good line for new artists since this pigment line requires more passes to saturate well in the skin, giving the artist the chance to slowly layer the pigment without the risk of over-saturation.

Organic pigment doesn't offer a room for messing up, the result can be much more permanent than inorganic pigment. They are very easily implanted in the skin and the artist is required to have a light hand to avoid over-saturation of the pigment. The best clients for this type of pigment are those who wish to have a fairly long-lasting (slower fading) pigmented brows and are committed to a specific color and shape. Oily and thick skin can benefit from organic pigment since it's easier to implement and slower to fade. It is crucial to pay attention to the depth of your blade using organic pigment; it will result in a long-term ashy/charcoal color migration in the skin. Tip: the artist can dilute the pigment for less concentrated pigmentation.

Golden Rule*

*Always be conservative with your application, regardless of the skin type or pigment type you are working with, **less is always better** and it is much easier to add than to reverse the process. We can always go with a darker color or make the shape thicker when clients come back for their initial touch-up. Have a gentle light pressure applied during the application; easier to go deeper once you know your* *client's skin after the initial healed results. Tell your client you are being conservative with your application in order to adjust as needed for the touch-up. Trust me, they will appreciate you for being careful with their face.*

PIGMENT ALLERGIES

There is no definitive evidence to suggest that organic pigments cause fewer allergies compared to inorganic pigments. Allergic reactions to permanent makeup pigments can occur with both organic and inorganic types, and the likelihood of an allergic reaction varies from person to person.

The risk of allergic reactions is influenced by individual factors such as skin sensitivity, personal medical history, and immune system responses. While some people may be more sensitive to certain organic pigments, others might react to specific inorganic pigments, too. Allergic reactions are relatively **rare** in permanent makeup procedures, but they can still happen. To minimize the risk of allergic reactions, especially if your client has a history of allergies (like topical makeup products, hair dyes, gold, silver, nickel) or sensitive skin, it is best to offer a patch test before the procedure, this can be done by creating a very small scratch on the skin (usually behind the ear) and apply a small amount of flesh pigment color or the chosen pigment to the scratch, and observe for any adverse reactions over a period of 72 hours. It is also very important to use high-quality pigments and follow proper hygiene and safety protocols to reduce the risk of complications during and after the procedure. Using nitrile gloves is highly recommended and latex-free materials to eliminate any potential risk of allergies.

It is also important to educate your clients about the proper personal hygiene during the healing period to avoid irritation or infections. (In depth in chapter 15)

MSDS (MATERIAL SAFETY DATA SHEETS)

Keeping a copy of Material Safety Data sheets, now known as Safety Date Sheets (SDS) for permanent pigments, is important for several reasons: Safety and health compliance, emergency response, regulatory compliance, ingredient information, and long-term reference.

1. SDS provides essential information about the potential hazards associated with the pigment, including information about the chemicals and substances used in its composition. This information is critical for ensuring the safety and health of individuals who handle or are exposed to the pigment.

2. In case of accidents, fires, spills, or other emergencies such as allergic reactions involving the pigment, having an up-to-date SDS readily available can be vital for first responders and emergency personnel. It helps them understand the nature of the materials involved and how to respond appropriately.

3. Regulatory agencies, such as OSHA (Occupational Safety and Health Administration) in the UNITED States, often require businesses and organizations to maintain SDS for hazardous chemicals and substances. Depending on your jurisdiction and industry, you may be legally obligated to have these documents on hand.

4. SDS contains detailed information about the chemical composition of the pigment, which can be valuable for various purposes, such as product labeling, handling, and understanding any potential long-term health risks associated with exposure.

5. Keeping SDS on hand ensures that you have access to important product information, including storage recommendations, safe handling procedures, and disposal guidelines. This knowledge helps you use and store the pigment, numbing agents, BARBICIDE, or any disinfecting solutions safely and efficiently.

6. In some cases, customers, suppliers, or regulatory authorities may request access to SDS as part of compliance checks, audits, or inquiries. Having the information available can expedite this process.

7. Pigments can be used in various applications, and you may need to refer to SDS even years after the initial purchase so keeping a copy ensures that you have access to this information whenever necessary.

It's important to keep your SDS up to date and make sure that they reflect any changes in the composition or safety information of the pigment. If you no longer use a particular pigment, you should still maintain the corresponding SDS for a reasonable period to meet potential future regulatory.

Eveline Benjamin

Chapter 7

BLADES

Blade sizes and how to choose the right one

BLADES

It's important to note that the choice of microblading blade size depends on factors such as the client's natural eyebrow hair, desired outcome, and your expertise. You may also use the combination of blade sizes, if need be, to achieve a natural-looking result. However, there are many types, shapes and sizes to choose from and it can get confusing, so allow me to simplify it for you.

Types

There are two main types of blades: hard blades and flexi blades (also called soft blades). What is the difference between the two?

1. Hard blades: They are made from high-quality medical-grade stainless steel and they are rigid. They have a fixed and hard structure, which means that the blade itself doesn't bend or flex during the microblading process and tends to go deeper in the skin. Because of their rigid nature, they require a steady and skilled hand to ensure accurate strokes and proper depth. Most suitable for thick, tough skin.

2. Flexi Blades: They are designed with a bit more flexibility in mind. These blades are made from high -quality medical-grade stainless steel. Flexi blades are often used for creating softer, more natural -looking strokes, as their flexibility can adapt to the contours of the skin more easily because the base absorbs some of the pressure and that helps the blade from penetrating the skin too deep. They are suitable for all skin types.

Sizes & Shapes

There are many sizes and shapes for blades on the market, and they are based on:

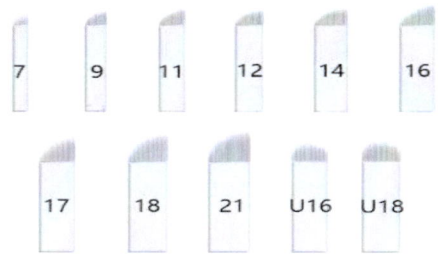

1. Needle count configuration, ranging from 7-21.

2. Needle diameter used in the configuration, ranging from 0.15-0.30.

3. The shape of the blade.

   - U-shape

   - Curved shape

   - Flat or slanted shape

Needle count: Is the number of needles (pins) in the blade and it directly correlates to the length of the strokes created; for example, a 7-9 needle configuration is usually used for short strokes which is required if you are working on thin brows or detailed work as in filling in between the main strokes vs. 14+ needle blade would be used for creating longer strokes in order to create thicker brows. 12 pin blade is a universal size that would create a medium-length stoke.

Needle diameter: Is the size of the needles used to create the blade, thin needles diameter creates fine strokes vs. thicker needles diameter create thicker strokes. Micro blades diameters are 0.18 mm | 0.20 mm | 0.25 mm| 0.30 mm, and Nano blades are 0.15 mm| 0.16 mm.

Needle shape: The most popular shapes used among artists are the U shape blade and the curved blade. Each shape helps you achieve curved strokes which is important in creating natural-looking brows. It really comes down to what you are comfortable working with and what helps you achieve the best-healed results. I personally favor the Flexi U-shape blade over all the others. The reason?

Realistically, U-shape blade makes two curved blades, so I am able to use both sides within the same procedure, just as if I would to use two new separate curved blades. Some blades can get dull during the procedure, especially if you are working on tough skin; doing so would 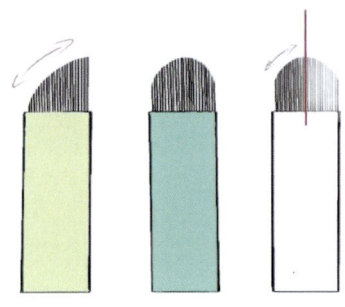 guarantee a clean cut into the skin by changing sides. Also, let's not forget to mention that it's cost-effective, two blades for the price of one during one session. It is also very important to know that you cannot use the upper tip of the U blade to create strokes, as it will create a jigged healed stroke line; only the sides of the blade can be used.

How To Choose The Right Blade For Your Client?

Due to the different sizes of blades available on the market, it is important to know which blade to use per client. The best way to figure this out is by running your own Q&A in your head.

- Does she have existing brow hair or nonexciting?

- The hair structure is it dense or fine?

- Does she have half-brow or full-on bulb to tails?

- Is her skin young or old?

- Is her skin thick or thin?

- Is her skin oily, normal, or dry?

In general, the right blade choice is based on your client's actual natural brow hair. If your client has a thick texture to her brow hair then a thicker blade would be much suited for a better blend with her natural; however, thin textured natural brow hair would require a thinner blade to blend in better with her soft natural brows she has. With that being said, you should always want to keep in mind that some strokes created in the skin can heal thicker in certain skin types, especially oily skin since it has the tendency to blur, so it is best to use one size slightly thinner at first until you are able to see the final healed results when your client come back for the initial touch-up, at that point you will be able to determine if a thicker blade is required or you could be counting your blessing at that point for taking a conservative approach right from the start when you see that your strokes have healed thicker.

Golden Rule*

It is best to involve your client in every choice making during the procedure; we have to respect the fact that it's their face we are working on, and their opinion and choices matter. Although they don't know much about the process and have zero knowledge about pigments and blades or the dos and don'ts, it is important to explain as the professional why you believe a specific pigment will suit them better than the other, and why this choice of blade would work better for their specific brow needs and the outcome they desire. Involving them guarantees happier clients, adds to their trust in your knowledge and an overall better understanding of the process with some reasonable and realistic expectations for the final results.

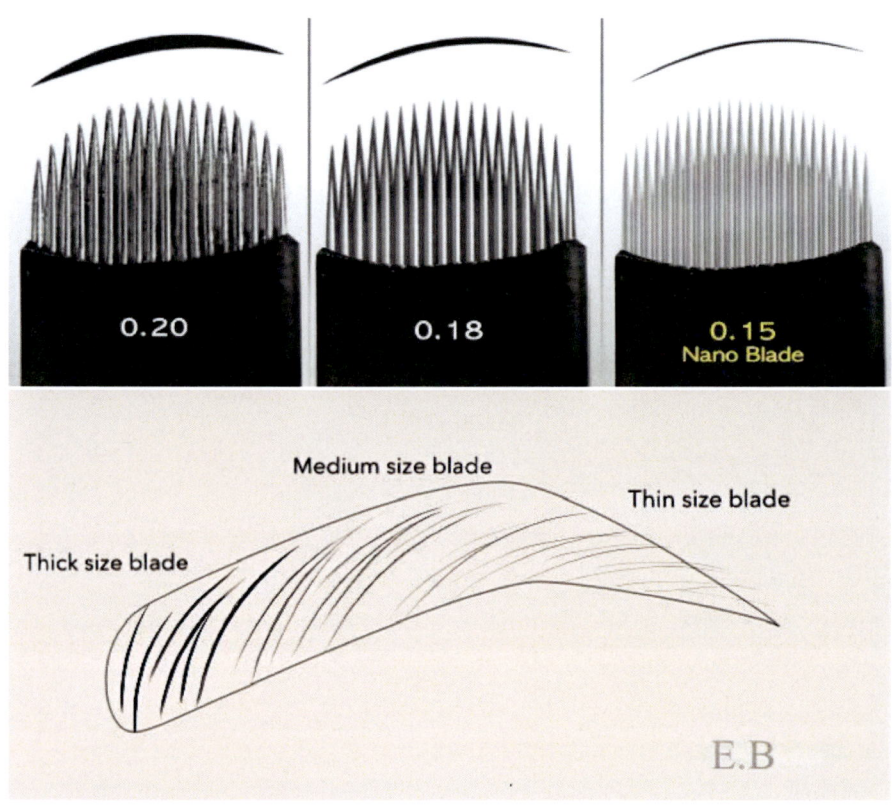

Let us start with:

1. **Hair texture and density, partially existing or non-existing brow hair.**

   - For clients with existing brow hair, you would need to match blade size with the texture and density of your client's existing brow hair strands. If your client has a thick, dense coarse hair strand, you would probably need to use a blade size 0.25 mm depending on how thick her natural is;

if she is more of a medium or medium-thick strand then you would need to use 0.20 mm, and if she has thin or medium-thin, a 0.18 mm or 0.20 mm. Use your best judgment based on what you see exists, and always remember that some strokes could heal thicker based on your client's unique skin.

- For clients with partial brows, missing the front or the tails, you can match her existing hair strand density with one of the micro blades to create your main strokes and then fill in between with nano tiny thin strokes to create a realism effect. For example, if her brow hair strand density matches well with blade size 0.25, use this size for main strokes and fill in a little with 0.18 mm or 0.16 mm nano in between.

- For clients with non-existing brow hair, you literally have the freedom to work your magic on a clean canvas and to create your own master piece of beautiful brows! However, don't get too excited yet! You still must take a few important considerations seriously before you

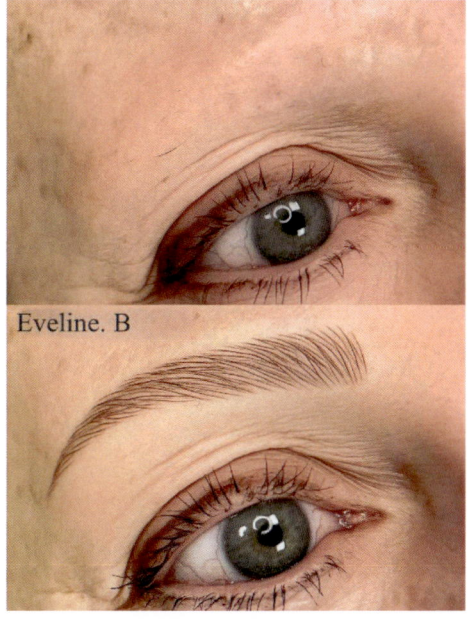

Eveline. B

become your own version of Picasso! ☺ Look at the overall picture when you look at your client; if she is older, then a softer brow look is a better option for her, and if she is a young-middle age lady then Microblading or the combo of Micro and Nano would create a beautiful set of brows for her. Also, check the density of their scalp hair, which will give you an idea of her previous natural brow hair density. Ask your client about how her brows looked before they were all gone and if she can provide you with an old photo of how they looked like naturally. The combination of micro and nano blades works great to create a realistic effect.

2. <u>Skin density and age.</u>

- <u>Older skin</u>: Older skin is more fragile, thinner, wrinkled and in general, more compromised by medication and/or environment. Avoid using hard type blades on older skin instead a flexi blade with a range of 0.16mm - 0.20 mm would work just fine, match blade diameter with her existing brow hair; if non-existing, a 0.18 mm is a good place to start until you see the initial healed result. The reason you would want to stick with thinner blades on older skin is due to their reduced elasticity and drier skin tendency; a thinner cut is less traumatizing to their skin and will still be capable to hold on to the pigment well since oil production is to the minimum, also, the stokes will heal faster. Keep in mind, thinner blades are sharper, so gliding softly over the skin should be enough to create the cut; if more pressure is required then you can do so as needed. The main focus should be on not going deep!

- <u>Younger skin</u>: The younger skin would obviously be much healthier and hydrated than older skin and in general their skin can handle all kind of blade types. Hard blades are good for thicker or tough skin vs medium to thinner or sensitive skin types a flexi blade type would be a better option. Choose the size of the blade based on the texture of their natural brow hair and the desired thickness of the shape to be created.

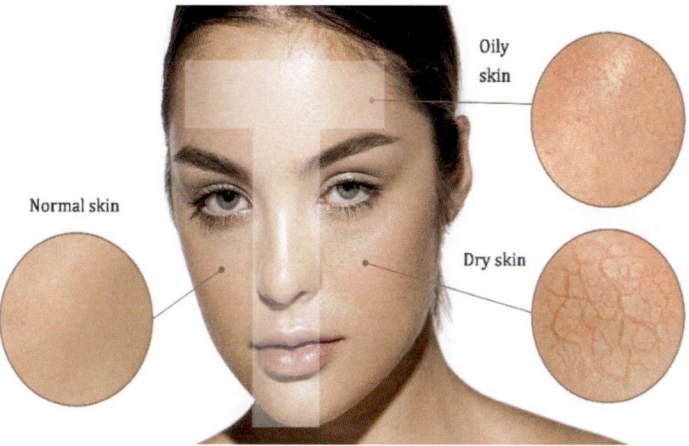

3. <u>Skin Function Type.</u>

- <u>Normal Type</u>

  Normal skin provides a stable canvas for PMU procedures, retaining pigment and the shape well, resulting in an excellent healing result. This type of skin is characterized by being well-balanced in terms of oil production, hydration, and texture. Here are some helpful common characteristics to help you identify normal skin:

  1. Normal skin has a moderate and balanced level of oil production.

  2. The texture of normal skin is generally smooth and even.

  3. Normal skin is adequately hydrated and retains moisture well. It neither feels excessively dry nor oily.

4. Pore size on normal skin is typically moderate. Neither enlarged nor too small.

5. The skin tone is relatively even and consistent. Normal skin doesn't have a lot of redness, irritation, or visible veins.

6. Normal skin is less reactive to certain products or environmental factors.

Any kind of blade shape or size would work great on this skin type, resulting in crisp, healed result with great pigment retention lasting on average for up to 18 months.

- Dry Type

  Although dry skin is not a great type of skin for any individual for the specific characteristic listed below, it is however, benefiting when it comes to PMU procedures. Microbladed hair strokes will heal very crisp and retain color for the longest amount of time among other skin types, on average 1.5+ years. Lacking normal oil production eliminates potential pigments dilution and therefore, the skin retains pigments well. Here are some helpful common characteristics to help you identify dry skin:

  1. Dry skin lacks proper hydration and often feels tight or less elastic. It may appear flaky, especially in areas prone to dryness.

  2. It can sometimes appear dull, lackluster, and may have a rough texture.

  3. Tends to develop fine lines and wrinkles more easily due to reduced natural oil production and moisture levels.

4. Dry skin is often sensitive and can be prone to irritation and redness, especially when exposed to harsh skincare products and environmental factors.

5. Pores on dry skin may appear smaller, but they can become more noticeable when skin is extremely dehydrated.

Flexi-type blades are most recommended for dry skin and pretty much a thinner blade size is preferred in this case since the skin is more fragile and lacks moisture as well as elasticity. However, on average, you can use 0.18 mm - 0.20 mm, depending on her natural brow hair texture.

- Combination Type

  Combination skin has characteristics of both oily and dry skin, with different areas of the face exhibiting varying levels of oiliness and dryness. Typically, the T-zone (forehead, nose, and chin) tends to be oilier which in a way, makes the skin on your brow area react to PMU brow procedure the same as Oily skin. Here are some helpful common characteristics to help you identify combination skin:

  1. The T-zone area might have more active oil glands, leading to a tendency for excess oily production and occasional breakouts.

  2. The cheeks and other areas might experience dryness, flakiness, and lack of moisture.

  3. Pores in the T-zone can be larger and more prone to becoming clogged, while pores in drier areas may appear smaller.

4. Combination skin can be sensitive in some areas, particularly the cheeks and areas prone to dryness.

5. Makeup application can be tricky due to the different textures of the skin. Products might not adhere well in oily areas and can emphasize dry patches in drier areas.

- Oily Type

   Oily skin is characterized by an overproduction of sebum, the skin's natural oil. This excess oil can lead to a very shiny appearance, enlarged pores and in increased likelihood of certain skin issues. It is important to note that the severity of these characteristics can vary from person to person. Here are some common characteristics of oily skin:

   1. Oily skin often appears shiny all over the face, especially in the T-zone area; therefore, combination skin is very similar to oily skin on how it impacts the results and longevity of microblading,

   2. Oily skin tends to have larger pores. These pores can become clogged with oil, dead skin cells, and impurities, leading to the formation of blackheads, whiteheads, and acne (pimples, pustules, and cysts).

   3. Makeup may have difficulty staying in place on oily skin due to the excess oil production, requiring touch-ups throughout the day.

Both combination skin and oily skin can present unique challenges when it comes to any PMU technique used to enhance the brows, and in both cases, these skin types can have an impact on the results and longevity of microblading. Let's go over some of the challenges:

1. Color retention: The excess oil can cause the pigment to spread and fade faster, leading to reduced color retention over time.

2. Blurred strokes: Excess oil can make the strokes appear softer, lighter, or less saturated. The fine lines can blur lighter, making the strokes less crisp and defined, and it can result in a more diffuse appearance of the strokes.

3. Fading and touch-ups: Clients with oily skin may require more frequent touch-up sessions compared to other skin types since the excess oil causes pigments to break down and fade faster.

4. Risk of infection: Oily skin can also be prone to acne and other skin issues. The risk of infection or complications may be slightly elevated, so proper aftercare and hygiene are crucial.

5. Aftercare challenges: The aftercare protocol is crucial for ensuring proper healing and color retention after microblading. Oily skin can make it more difficult for the skin to heal properly, as excessive oil production can interfere with the healing process. The best after care for oily skin is to use the dry-healing approach. (More details in aftercare chapter-15)

Remember that individual results can vary, and while oily skin might present some challenges, many people with oily skin have successfully undergone microblading and achieved beautiful results.

The only question remains now is, what type of blade is best suited for such challenging skin?

Matching blade size with the actual hair strand still applies in this case; however, the fact that strokes are more likely to blur and heal thicker should never be ignored either, so sticking with a thinner blade than the actual hair texture is the safest approach for the initial procedure until you can assess the healed result on their touch up appointment. Depending on the natural texture of their brow hair, I personally like to start with 0.18 mm, I know it's thin but again, I need to see how that stroke heals before I venture to a thicker one if needed, a 0.20 mm or a 0.25 mm should be your next size up but definitely no larger than 0.25mm.

Furthermore, and most importantly, apply fewer strokes and depending on your blade size, leaving an average of 2-3 mm of negative space between strokes is very important to avoid migration; as mentioned previously once you assess the initial healed result, you can decide how to adjust the application.

There are mixed opinions about what is the best PMU application for oily skin. Here is my personal opinion based on my many years in PMU field.

- Many believe in and promote machine strokes (Nano Brows), machine method of application is a doted motion as the needle penetrates the skin to implement the pigment in the skin, deeper and more saturated, creating more of a permanent application.

- Many believe Ombre is the best technique for oily skin, which is more of a solid makeup look; I personally agree that it is a good option indeed if your client prefers that look.

- Some promotes Micro-shading (a combination of strokes and powdery shading style or ombre style combined). I've seen many who have had it done and it honestly heals into a full Ombre eventually.

- Others like myself still believe that blading is still the safest method of application for oily skin and for one main reason: for the shallow strokes to blur and completely fade fast is a much better problem to deal with than if they were to blur and smudge into an ashy looking puddle for many years.

My advice is to always take extra precautions when working on oily skin; we can never 100% predict the healed results on any skin type as is,

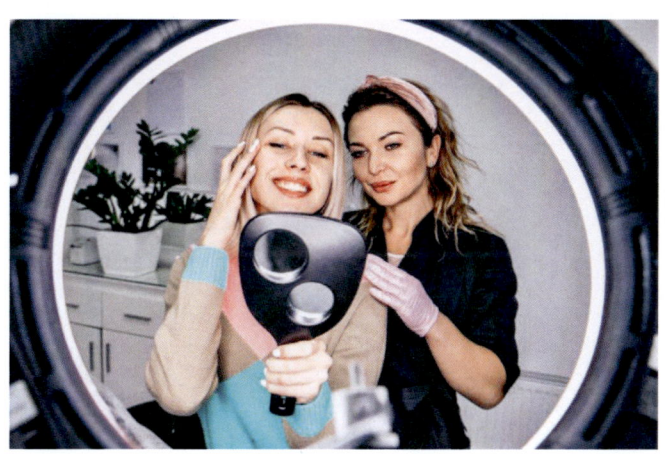

and more so with oily skin. The conservative approach is definitely the key factor in this case.

Just remember, the goal is for your client to be extremely happy and pleased with the final result.

Happy clients, happy us!

WHEN AND HOW TO USE MANUAL SHADING WHILE KEEPING THE NATURAL MICRO-BLADED LOOK?

Shading, also called pixelization, it's created using a dotting motions method, either by a manual tool similar to microblading tool or a machine. Manual shading is a technique used to complement microblading results by filling in between strokes or sometimes used to create a fully shaded brow-like ombre, lightest on the inner part of the brow and gradually darkens gradually towards the tail.

In this manual, the main focus is obviously on how to create natural fluffy-looking brows using blading method without shading; however, learning the manual shading technique can be useful sometimes and in certain cases, your client might desire that final makeup look so it is good to be familiar with the technique. Manual shading is an easy technique in comparison to machine shading technique. Learning machine PMU work can be difficult; it requires a lot of time to practice and to perfect the technique in order to achieve successful result without messing up. It should be definitely the next course up after learning manual application but not before; I believe a lot of ethical instructors would agree with this fact.

It is important to know that machine shading is more permanent, and the same applies to manual shading if done too deeply; therefore, if you don't intend to create permanent shading and just enough to enhance the overall look, make sure your application is very shallow by tapping/dotting gently in the areas you want to fill. Shading is always done after microblading and between strokes to create a subtle shade between them. It is very much suitable to neutralize and color correct old tattoos, or people with partial brows to create a full even flow in alignment with existing hair, or even between far-apart strokes done on oily skin with no existing hair to fill in some of the big gaps, also, it's crucial to make sure it's very shallow and light application as you want to create more of semi-shading than permanent-shading, mainly to have the strokes and shading fade gradually at the same pace. You want to focus on the center of the brows or the center of the strokes to create a subtle enhancement without too much of overlapping as shown below. Shading needles are available in many shapes and sizes, as shown below.

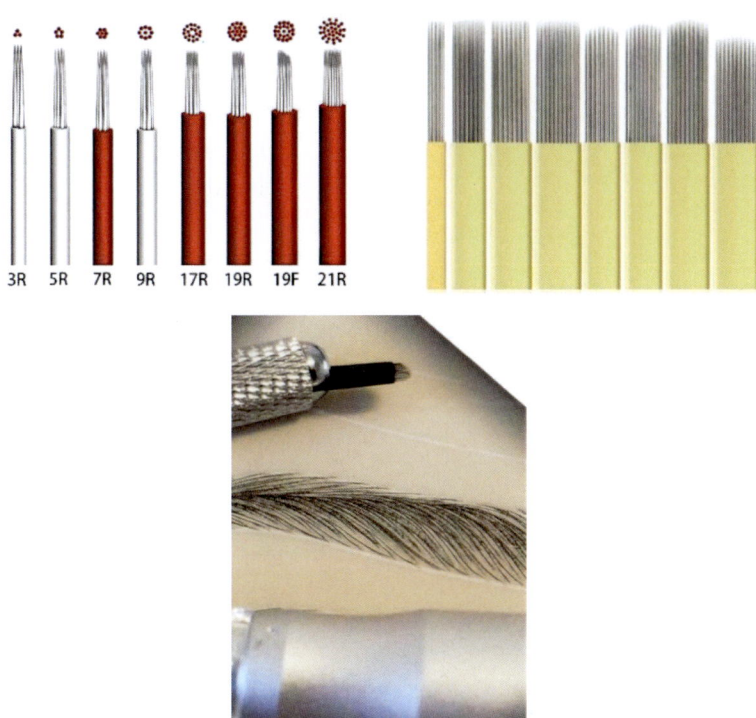

Flat shaders - They are used for outlining brow shape and for shading in narrow areas such as the tail of the brow or between strokes. Since they are flat and narrow, they fit nicely into tight spaces.

Double row shaders - Double row shaders are designed with 2 straight rows of flat needles (pins). This style can be used in narrow and wider areas of the brow to shade throughout.

Round shaders - round shaders are an all-around great shading tool. Use a larger grouping of needles (pins) in larger areas of shading to implant more pigment at a faster rate for a better and more disbursed shading effect and less trauma to the skin. Use a smaller grouping of needles (pins) for smaller areas of shading, such as the tail arch or a very thin brow shape. Single needles or 3-needle shaders are great for lightly shading the bulb area or for the pointillism effect.

HOW TO READ YOUR BLADE MANUFACTURER SEALED POUCH?

When you purchase your blades, they will come sealed in their manufactures sealed pouch and on the back of the pouch, you will see all the checked boxes in reference to the blade. For example, as you see below, this specific blade size is 0.18 mm, it is the Flexy type and configuration (pin count) is 7. It is also important to keep an eye on the Exp date; the blade is a little dull after the expiration date and will not perform well. There are many companies out there that sell different kinds of blades, some are one-piece (blade already attached to the handle) completely disposable and some are individually wrapped blades for you to manually attach to a separate handle.

A one-unit handle piece is more expensive and if the blade has some kind of a default, then the whole piece is in the trash, on average $8 per unit. On the other hand, if you decide to invest in individually wrapped blades, they are cheaper depending on the source chosen.

DISPOSABLE. STERILE. SINGLE USE ONLY

MICROBLADING NEEDLE
(316STAINLESS STEEL) Dia (mm)
0.25☐ 0.20☐ 0.18☑ 0.16☐

☑7P	☐21P	☐19U		☐19RL
☐V	☐9P	☐12U	☐21U	☐21RL
☑Flexy	☐12P	☐14U	☐3RL	☐9M
☐Hard	☐14P	☐16U	☐5RL	☐15M
☐Shade	☐16P	☐17U	☐9RL	☐17M
	☐18P	☐18U	☐17RL	☐19M

CE ISO STERILE EO ②

Exp Date:11.15.2024

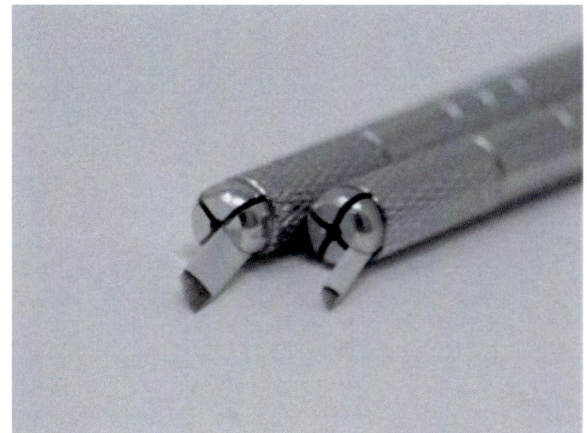

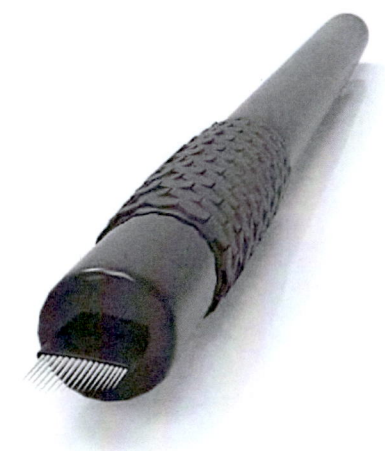

Eveline Benjamin

Chapter 8

FACE SHAPE, EYE SHAPE

Understanding face shapes, eye shapes and brow styles

FACE SHAPES

The shape of the face can influence the choice of eyebrow shape that complements people's features. It is essential to consider not only the individual face shape but also their personal style and the natural shape of their existing eyebrows when choosing a brow shape that is most flattering for their own unique features.

Here are some general guidelines for selecting the right eyebrow shape based on the facial shape:

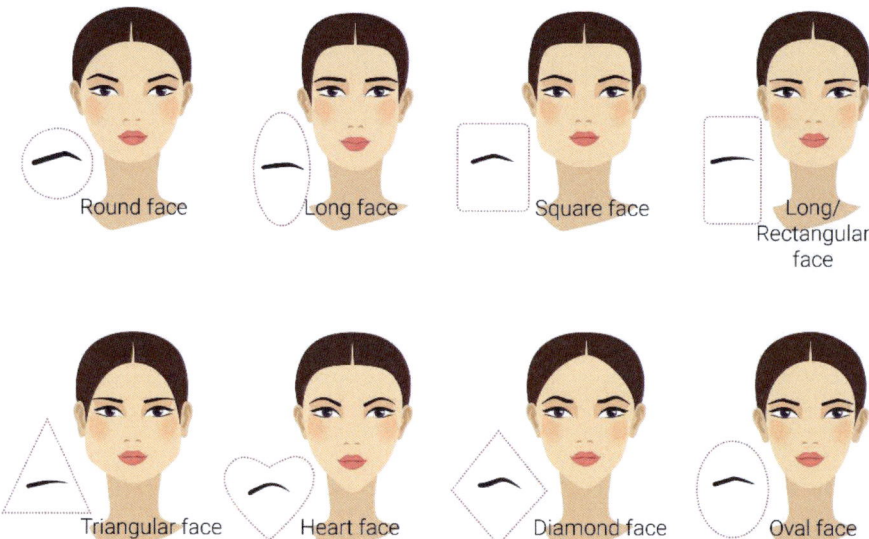

1. **Round face:** Brow shape: Angular and slightly arched eyebrows can help add definition to a round face. High, well-defined arches can make the face appear longer and slimmer.

2. **Long /Rectangular face:** Brow shape: A flatter, horizontal brow shape can visually shorten the face. Avoid overly high or arched brows, as they can make the face appear longer.

3. **Square face**: Brow shape: Soften the angles of a square face with slightly rounded or softly arched brows. Avoid overly angular or harshly shaped brows, as they can emphasize the squareness.

4. **Oval Face:** Brow shape: oval faces are versatile and can work with various brow shapes. A soft, natural arch often complements an oval face shape well.

5. **Heart shape:** Brow shape: A rounded or slightly curved brow shape can complement a wider forehead and narrower chin of a heart-shaped face. Avoid overly thin or high-arched brows.

6. **Diamond face:** Brow shape: Softly curved or rounded brows can balance the angularity of a diamond-shaped face. Avoid overly sharp or pointed arches.

7. **Triangular face or Pear-shaped face:** Brow shape: Balance the broader forehead of a triangular face with softly arched brows. These brows can help draw attention away from the forehead.

8. **Long face:** Brow shape: A flatter, horizontal brow shape with and outer very soft arch can visually shorten the face. Avoid high-arched brows, as they can make the face appear much thinner and longer.

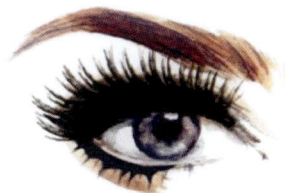 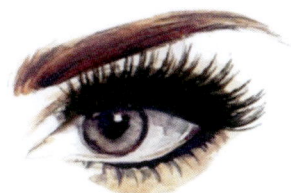

The best brow shape for an individual often depends on their unique facial features and personal preferences. However, there are some general guidelines as we know for selecting a brow shape that complements different eye shapes as well. Here are some recommendations:

- **Round eyes**: For round eyes, go for slightly arched brows. The arch can help elongate the eyes and create the illusion of almond-shaped eyes.

- **Almond eyes**: Almond-shaped eyes are already quite balanced, so a soft, natural arch can work well. Avoid overly dramatic or angular shapes.

- **Hooded eyes**: If you are working on hooded eyes, you can create the illusion of larger eyes with slightly arched brows. A higher arch can help lift the appearance of the eyes and make them look more open.

- **Monolid eyes**: Go for a straight or a slight upward slope with a soft arch and short tails to help open the eyes.

- **Close-set eyes**: To visually balance close-set eyes, a wider gap between the eyebrows can help. Keep the brows more horizontal and avoid a high arch.

- **Wide-set eyes**: For wide-set eyes, a slightly closer brow can create a more balanced look. Try a slightly higher arch to draw attention towards the center of the face.

- **Deep-set eyes**: With deep-set eyes, a medium to high arch can work well. It can help bring more attention to the eyes and create a lifting effect.

- **Upturned eyes**: These eyes have a natural upward slant. Go for a more horizontal or softly rounded brow shape to balance the eye shape.

- **<u>Downturned eyes</u>**: Downturned eyes have a natural droop at the outer corners. A lightly upturned brow with a higher arch can help lift the eyes and counteract the downturned look.

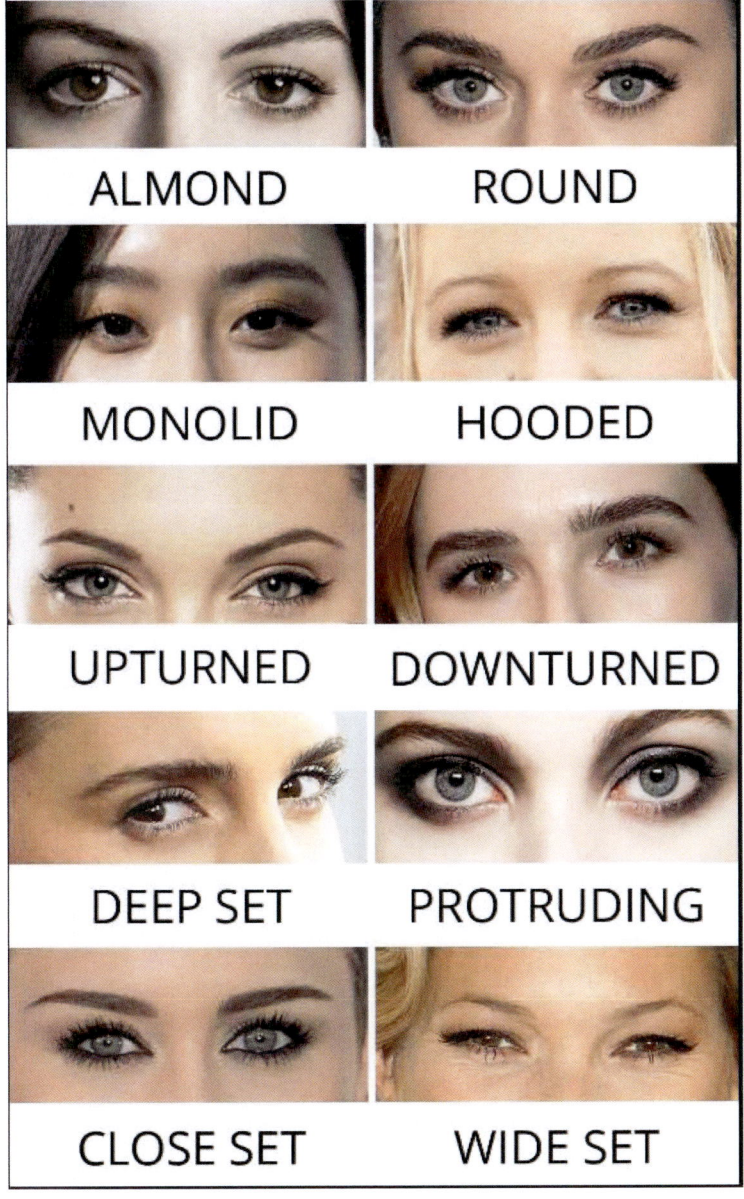

Eveline Benjamin

Chapter 9

BROW MEASUREMENT

&

MAPPING

MEASUREMENTS & MAPPING

To create natural-looking eyebrows, precise measurements and careful planning are essential. The initial steps involve measuring and marking key points to determine the ideal shape and placement of the brows using the facial golden ratio, also known as the "beauty golden ratio" or "phi mask," this is a mathematical concept that suggests there are ideal facial proportions that are considered more attractive or beautiful. It's derived from the golden ratio (Phi), and it is used in various fields, including art, fashion, and plastic surgery, to determine what is considered a harmonious and attractive facial structure to achieve aesthetically pleasing proportions.

In relation to brow design, most makeup artists and PMU professionals use the golden ratio as a guideline to create balanced and harmonious eyebrows. The ideal brow shape and proportion can vary from person to person, but the golden ratio can be a helpful starting point and the key aspect is to aim for a balanced and natural look.

The golden ratio in relation to brow design suggests the following:

1. Start point: The starting point of the brow should align with the inner corner of the eye. If you were to draw an imaginary line from the inner corner of the eye to the forehead, it would help define the starting point of the eyebrow.

2. Arch point: The highest point of the arch should be around two-thirds of the way from the start point to the end point of the eyebrow.

3. End point: The end point of the eyebrow should align with a line drawn from the outer corner of the eye to the outer edge of the nose.

Brow shape preferences can vary among individuals, and personal preferences play a significant role in determining the final outcome of brow design; always consult with your clients to understand their preferences and ensure that the brow shape you create aligns with their desired look and complements their facial features.

Another important point is symmetry; ensuring that the eyebrows are symmetrical is crucial. Measuring and comparing the distance between various points on both eyebrows to ensure balance. The goal is to create brows that look like a better version of the client's natural eyebrows by following the golden ration while still keeping in consideration of their own unique facial features and bone structure.

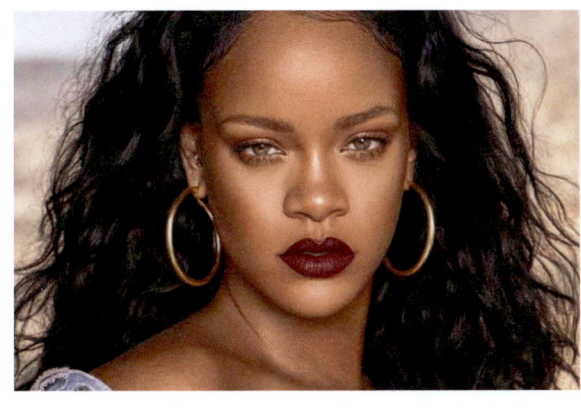

Remember that while the golden ratio can serve as a useful guideline, it's not a strict rule. It's crucial to consider the individual's unique facial features and bone structure when designing their eyebrows. Not everyone's face conforms precisely to the golden ratio, so some adjustments may be necessary to achieve the most flattering and natural look.

Where and what you need to start:

Important Mapping Points

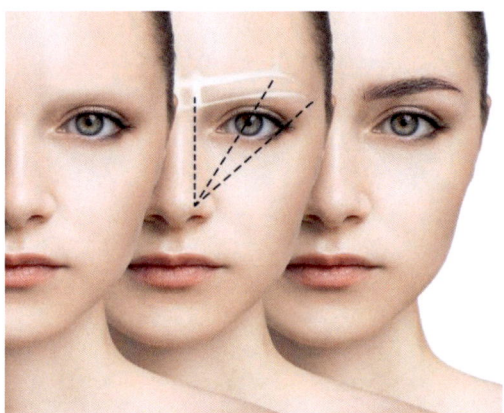

1. Start point

2. Arch point

3. End point

4. Thickness

5. Symmetry

6. Facial anatomy/bone structure

Important tools for mapping

1. Brow measuring ruler (any kind)

2. Mapping string (pre-inked)

3. Brow pencil (waterproof)

Important Points to Remember Before You Start Mapping

- Refresh both yours and your client's memory about what you discussed during the initial consultation.

- Go over the proper brow shape with her again and make sure she is still on the same page.

- Double-check with her that she did not sneak in a few units of Botox since her initial consultation visit.

- Have your client lay down with her eyes closed when you start with the measurement; it's important for their facial muscle to be relaxed to achieve a symmetrical outline.

- When the shape is drawn, have your client sit up to assess symmetry and the shape. Have your client do a few facial expressions to make sure all is aligned.

- Final step is getting her approval and adjusting the shape as needed per her request if need be.

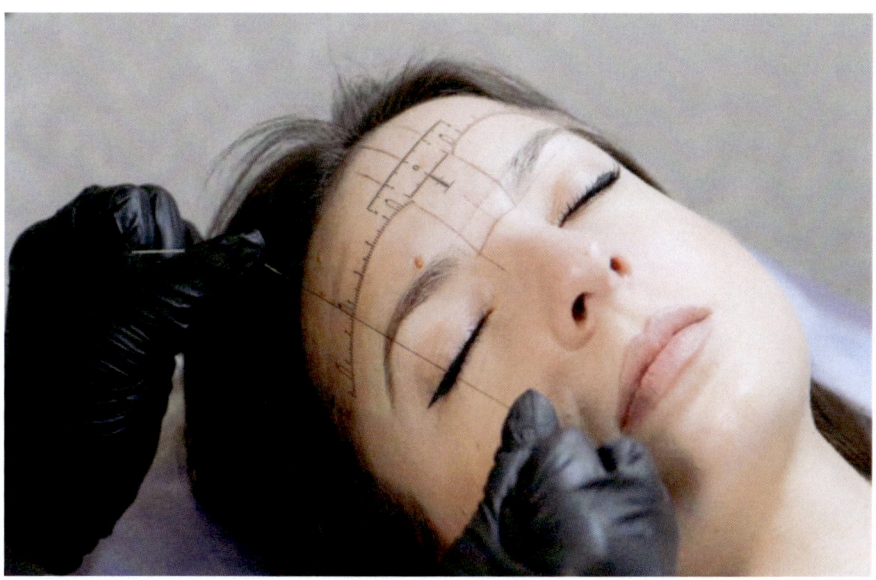

BROW MAPPING GENERAL RULE

Outlining the brows accurately before microblading ensures that the final results are symmetrical, well-proportioned, and aligned with the clients' desired look and with their existing features. Here are the steps to outline the brows (more in "procedure step by step chapter-14")

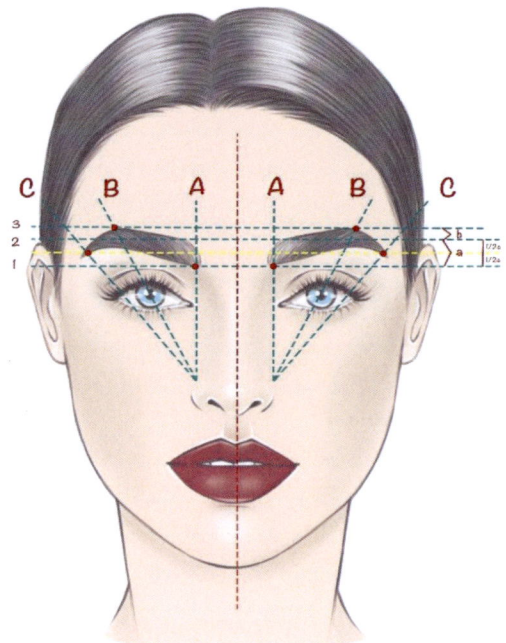

1. <u>Assess the client's face</u>

    Analyze the client's face shape, bone structure, and existing brow shape. Consider any asymmetries and areas that may need correction or enhancement.

2. <u>Place the ruler against the client's face to establish key reference points for the brows.</u>

    - <u>Starting point</u>: Align the ruler with the inner corner of the eye, going upward to find the starting point of the brow. Mark it lightly with a brow pencil. If your clients have wide-set eyes, then find your start point by creating your line from the inner bridge of their nose and mark your point.

- Arch point: Diagonally from the edge of the nose over the center of the pupil to find the highest point of the arch and mark it. You can also use the diagonal line to the outside of the iris if an outer arch is more flattering based on her facial structure and features especially for clients with long face shape.

- End point: Align the ruler with the edge of the nose over the outer corner of the eye to determine the endpoint and mark it.

- Thickness: The starting point is where you would need to determine the thickness of the brow design. Mark where the natural bottom hair start point line is, if any exists and right above it by 1 cm or less, this of course varies from one client to another based on their natural start and thickness of their brow and their preference on how thick or thin they want the brow to be. Adjust the height of the bottom starting point as you see suited, avoid giving her the grumpy or angry look.

3. Create the shape

Using the marked reference points, connecting them by drawing the upper and lower outlines of the brow using a brow pencil. Ensure the shape is symmetrical and balanced.

- Bottom of head and bottom of tail should run parallel.

- Arch should slope diagonally from the bottom center of forehead to the top of arch.

4. Consult with the client again.

Show the client the shape created and measurements, and discuss any adjustments or preferences they may have. Make sure the client is comfortable with the proposed outline. Keep in mind what you foresee of your design is something your client cannot envision, the lines will scare them a little so it is important for you to explain that the lines are just your guide and you will be mainly filling the inside area in between the lines, also, drawing few strokes with a marker inside your guidelines can help them understand it better. This step requires a bit of patience on your end because your client is at the point of giving their final ok before you start the procedure; they are nervous, and rightfully so.

CHALLENGING BROWS

Measuring and marking specific points on the face to create a balanced and symmetrical eyebrow shape on a symmetrical face is way easier than an asymmetrical brow challenge. Typically, it's one brow higher than the other, but sometimes along with that, you can be dealing with a brow extremely rounder or flatter than the other or a previous faded tattoo that can limit you, and if it's your lucky day, your client can have a crooked nose that will just add more to the challenge in creating a harmonious balance. This is when you take a deep breath and focus on what can be done to enhance what she has while accepting your limited options. Communicate with your client and go over the only three options you can try to work with on her brows.

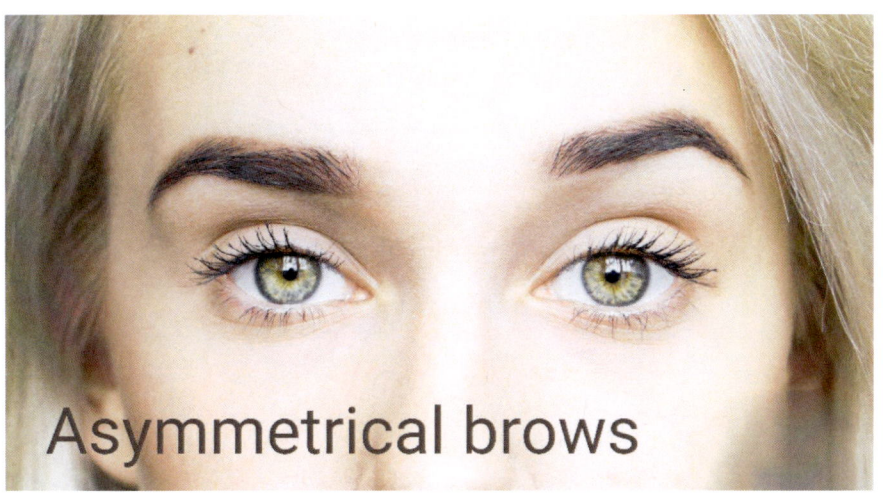

Asymmetrical brows

1. If you feel it's a muscle issue, suggest she goes for ½ or 1 unit of Botox into the Frontalis muscle above the brow; it can relax the brow downward and fix the issue before the procedure.

2. If it is a bone structure issue, you can adjust the brows slightly by removing some brow hair (top hair on higher brow) and some off (bottom of lower brow). It is important your client approves of this option before proceeding; furthermore, show her exactly where the hair will be removed to enhance the final look of the brows.

3. If option 1 and 2 are not good options for the client, then explain to her that the alignment cannot be improved, and all you can do at this point is give her a better brow shape and a fuller brow look; however, she would need to understand that by agreeing to doing so, the more defined and yet still asymmetrical brows will be more pronounced on her face and she might not like the final result. Your client should be willing to meet you halfway, understanding certain circumstances at play in her case. Your need to understand that you are not a miracle worker!

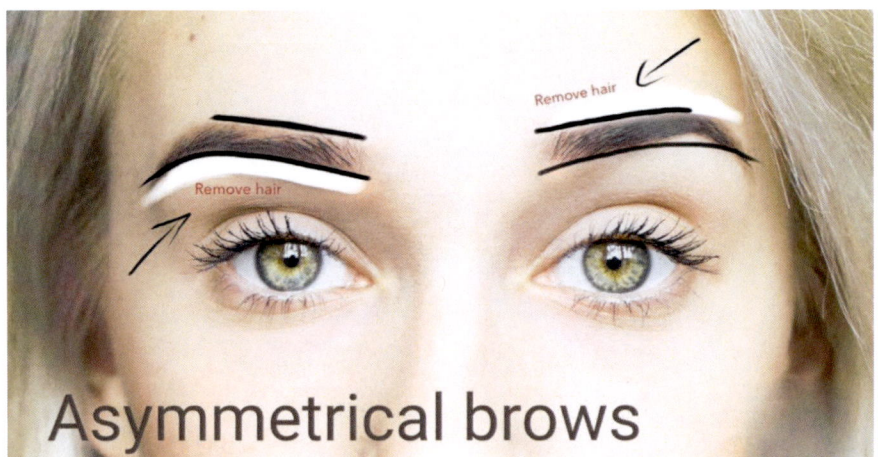

Asymmetrical brows

Chapter 10

CONSULTATION

&

CHARTING

Build a long-term client relation through integrity and professionalism

CONSULTATION

Consultations are an important initial step to ensure that the client is a good candidate for the procedure and to build a trusting client-artist relationship. It's a fundamental step in the process of providing the desired brow enhancement while ensuring a safe and satisfying experience for your client. It is best to provide your clients with all the forms prior to the consultation via email or a link to your digital forms. Ask your client to fill them out and bring the health history and consent form with them on their consultation appointment. It is never a good idea to schedule the initial consultation on the day of the procedure, just in case the client is not a good candidate for the procedure; that would be a few blocked hours on the schedule gone to waste.

✓ A consultation allows us to understand the clients' specific needs and expectations. Both you and your client can discuss the desired brow shape, thickness, color, and overall style to ensure your client's vision is clear.

✓ Microblading is not a one-size-fits-all procedure. Each client's brows are unique, and a consultation helps you tailor the procedure to the client's individual characteristics and preferences.

✓ It provides the opportunity to choose the right pigment color for your client; otherwise, if you are tight on time, you can do this step on the day of the procedure. Explain to your client that the pigment will need to match her natural eyebrow hair for it to look natural, not her scalp hair, and the fact that you will be involving her in the color choice so that you both are on the same page.

✓ Naturally, your client will have questions and concerns about the procedure, process, pain, healing time, aftercare, the fear of eyebrow hair loss and the final outcome; respect their concerns, be informative and answer thoroughly. After all, it is their face and you want to make sure they are aware of all pros and cons before they make their final decision. Note: microblading is a superficial application and has no negative effect on existing brow hair.

✓ The consultation is an opportunity to go over your client's medical history, any allergies, and potential contraindications; these issues may affect the suitability of microblading. Based on her health condition and your concerns, it is also your opportunity to ask your client to obtain a written note or to request a doctor's authorization to be emailed to you in order to perform the procedure. Make sure it's a legitimate note!

✓ Manage their expectations, explain that microblading is a semi-permanent procedure, the results will fade overtime, and potential touch-ups are required to keep the brows looking good. You also need to inform them that microblading is meant to give a natural brow look on a daily basis and will not provide the makeup filled-in look; they will probably need to fill them in slightly when they apply their full makeup. If they require more of a filled-in makeup look, shading will help with achieving that.

✓ Also, you want to explain to your client that results vary from one individual to another, explaining that their skin type, skin condition, environmental factors, lifestyle, internal factors, and how they take care of their brows plays a big role on how their brows will retain the pigment and the length of retention. "No guarantees should be given on your end about the final outcome other than your proper method of application. You are liable for what you deliver (proper application, proper design, and the right color per her approval) but not on how your client chooses to care and maintain her new micro-bladed brows".

✓ Go over pre-procedure information to prepare them for what they need to avoid prior to the procedure, explain that if they get a headache, Tylenol is a better option than Ibuprofen which thins the blood, and/or that amazing glass of wine a few days prior to the procedure could lead to more pinpoint bleeding during the procedure which has the potential to negatively affect the final healed color.

✓ Conduct yourself in a very professional manner yet keep friendly and sincere. Be informative, and understanding to help them feel more at ease and assure them that nothing can be done without their approval throughout the whole procedure.

It is important to establish a strong and trusting relationship with your client as it is vital to your success.

Charting

It is very important to <u>document</u> the procedure in your client's file, what you discussed, the choices given and what your client agreed on; it's essential for legal and professional purposes. Taking <u>before and after photos</u> is very crucial; some artists take a photo of the design with the client's thumbs up, indicating she is approving of it. Have a form stating potential changes to existing brows with multiple options to be checked and have your client sign it before starting the procedure. Make sure your client hands you a completed and signed health history and consent form if she hasn't already. You always want to cover yourself from some possible future disagreement. As an artist in this field or in any beauty service industry, for all it matters, we are liable for the final outcome of what we deliver. Therefore, documentation is important, not only if there's future dispute, it serves you to remember what was done and why for any given client of yours. Document;

- What blade you used.

- What pigment (brand, color and the formula if you mixed colors).

- Her skin's reaction (reactive, amount of bleeding, fluid oozing, or if there was a stubborn section not absorbing the pigment well).

- Add that she was part of the color & shape choice.

- State that she understands that you are being conservative with your initial application until you are able to assess her skin and healed results when she is back for the touch-up.

- Mention that you went over the aftercare with her in detail and to the best of your knowledge, she understood all the instructions and was given a chance to the ask questions.

- State that you explained the healing stages. That you gave her the aftercare healing ointment/cream/gel or if you instructed the dry healing method.

- Mention that she provided you with a doctor's note if you requested one based on her health condition.

- Note the healed results when she comes back for the touch-up and what was discussed and done to improve the shape or the color.

(Although it might take some extra time of your day, charting is something you will be thankful for, especially if you have a challenging memory like mine and when you have a huge number of clientele to work on).

Don't Do It!!!

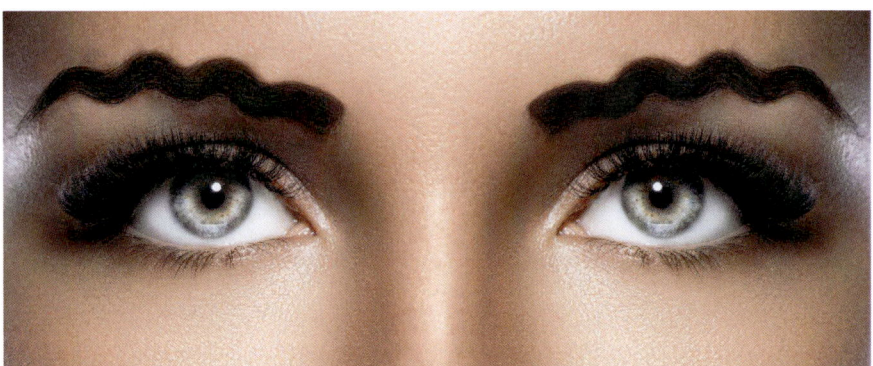

If you, as a PMU artist, do not agree with your client's desired brow shape, it's crucial to handle the situation professionally and ensure clear communication. Here are some steps to follow:

1. Start by **listening** to your client's preferences and understanding their desired brow shape. Ask them to explain what they have in mind and why they want that specific shape.

2. As a professional, you need to offer your **expert opinion** while being respectful of your client's wishes. If you believe the client's desired shape may not be the most flattering or suitable for her facial features, explain your concerns and provide alternatives that would work better.

3. Show **examples**, use reference photos or sketches to illustrate your suggested brow shape. This visual aid can help the client better understand your perspective and make an informed decision.

4. Explain how **her face shape** can influence the ideal brow shape. Different face shapes may benefit from specific brow styles, and

you can discuss how the suggested shape aligns with her unique features.

5. If the client is still insisting on a particular brow shape that you believe may not be the best choice, try to find a **compromise**. Perhaps you can meet halfway by adjusting the shape slightly to maintain a more natural appearance.

6. Ensure that the client fully understands and consents to the chosen brow shape. **Have them sign a consent** form that includes a description of the agreed-upon shape and color.

7. **Document it**! It's essential to document the conversation, including the client's final decision.

Remember that your client's satisfaction is crucial, but your expertise is also essential in achieving the best possible results. Don't be afraid to say **no** to a client; at the end of the day, she is a walking billboard of your work and a bad job or shape will affect your reputation, people's trust, and the success of your business. Open and respectful communication is key to finding a solution that both you and your client can be comfortable with, and if you feel that it's impossible then I urge you to advise her to go to a different artist who might share the same taste.

Chapter 11

SAMPLE FORMS

Health history form

Consent form

Pre-Procedure form

Aftercare form

Tools consent form

Healing stages sheet

Authorization to correct form

Chart

These are sample forms, for the purpose to be used as a reference in creating your own individual forms

SEMI-PERMANENT MAKEUP HEALTH HISTORY FORM

Semi-Permanent Cosmetics (tattooing), Microblading/ Nano-Blading/Nano Brows/ are invasive procedures that requires a thorough medical history. Please complete this questionnaire.

Name _____Age _____ DOB _____

Address_____

Telephone # _____ Email _____

Emergency contact _____ Telephone # _____

Are you currently under the care of a physician? If so, why?

_____

_____

_____

Do you have allergies to <u>Lidocaine</u> products? _____ Yes _____ No

Have you had any previous permanent makeup procedure? _____ Yes _____ No

If yes, please specify: _____

Are you <u>pregnant or breastfeeding</u>? _____ Yes _____ No

Have you used <u>Accutane</u> within the last 6-12 months? _____ Yes _____ No

Important***PLEASE LIST ALL ALLERGIES & MEDICATIONS:

_____

_____

_____

It is Red Cross policy that you cannot donate blood for one year from date of this procedure. If you have had hepatitis in the last 12 months you cannot have this procedure.

Skin History /Medications Health History

__Skin Cancer *	__Anti-Depressants	__Good __Poor
__Moles* - __Rosacea*	__Chemotherapy* Dr. Perm	__Alopecia
__Psoriasis*	__Radiation*area _____	__Heart Problems
__Bruise Easily	__Aspirin	__Arthritis
__Heals Normal - __ Delayed	__Blood Thinners*over 1mg	__Pregnant/Nursing*
__Use Retin A	__Pain Pills/Shots/steroids	__Cancer*
__Chemical Peel* 6w	__Tranquilizers*	__Hepatitis
__Cortisone Creams*	__Insulin	__HIV Virus
__Scars* - __Keloids*	__Anti-Herpes Med	__Lupus*
__Laser Therapy* 6w	__Vit E/ Fish Oil	__Diabetes*50/50
__Tattoo Removal		__Alcohol/Drug Abuse*
__Cosmetic Surgery* 6m		Seizures/Dizziness*50/50

SIGNATURE_____ DATE_____

MICROPIGMENTATION INFORMED CONSENT

Name: _____ Date of Birth: _____

Address: _____

City: _____ State: _____ Zip: _____

Cell Phone: _____ Home Phone: _____

Email Address: _____

How did you hear about us? (circle) Google / Facebook / Instagram / Yelp / Other / Referral (name) _____

The nature and method of the proposed semi-permanent makeup (cosmetic tattoo) procedure have been explained to me as having the usual risks inherent in the procedure and the possibility of complications during and following its performance. I understand that there may be a certain amount of discomfort or pain associated with the procedure and that other possible adverse side effects may include: minor and temporary bleeding, bruising, redness or other discoloration and/or swelling. Fading or loss of pigment may occur. Secondary infection in the area of the procedure is rare if properly cared for but may occasionally occur.

By signing below, I specifically acknowledge that I have been advised of the facts and matters set below, and I agree as follows:

(Please initial the line next to the number after you clearly understand each statement)

1. _____ I have informed the practitioner of any and all of my known allergies. I acknowledge that it is not always reasonably possible to determine in advance whether I might have an allergic reaction to any of the pigments, dyes, topical preparations, or processes used in the procedure, and I agree to accept the risk that such reaction is possible.

2. _____ I acknowledge that complications as a result of semi-permanent makeup procedures may occur, particularly in the event that the post-procedural instructions are not followed, and accept full responsibility for such complications.

3. _____ I realize that my body is unique and neither **(your business name)** or its employee can predict how my skin may react as a result of the procedure

nor can predict how well my skin will retain the pigment nor the length of retention.

4a. _____ I have previously had micropigmentation performed by someone other than **(your business name)** on the same area (brows) that I am asking **(your business name)** employee to work on today

____YES ____NO

4b. _____ IF YES, I understand that correcting or touching up micropigmentation that was performed by others involves additional risks because of the existence of permanent pigments of unknown composition, brand, color, age, shape and other factors over which **(your business name)** and its employee has no control. I understand that additional appointments after the initial and follow-up appointments may be required and will be billed at **(your business name)** standard rates. I understand that **(your business name)** cannot predict the results in advance and cannot guarantee and has not represented that the results will be as I desire. I understand and fully accept the risks associated with this procedure and hold **(your business name)** harmless from same.

5. _____ I acknowledge that the procedure may result in a long-lasting (few years) change to my appearance and that no guarantee has been given to me to the ability to later change or remove the results.

6. _____ I understand that future skin-altering procedures such as laser treatments, plastic surgery, Botox, and/or injections may alter and degrade my semi-permanent makeup and that I must inform any future service provider that I have had micropigmentation applied. I understand and accept that such changes are not the fault of **(your business name)** and its employees. I further understand that such changes or degradation in my appearance may not be correctable through further semi-permanent makeup procedures.

7. _____ I consent to the admittance of authorized observers to the procedure(s) for the purpose of education or assistance.

8. _____ I acknowledge that obtaining the semi-permanent makeup is my choice alone, and I consent to the procedure and to its attendant risks and to any actions or conduct of **(your business name)** and its employee reasonably necessary to perform the procedure.

9. _____ I understand that I will have the opportunity, within the time constraints of my appointment, to approve the design and color of the semi-permanent makeup to be applied, and I accept responsibility for same.

10. _____ I consent to any relevant photographs being taken both before and after the procedure to document the results of the procedure strictly for the internal use of **(your business name)**.

11. _____ [Optional/Requested] I consent to **(your business name)** using of my brow "before & after" photos of me for marketing purposes to display its capabilities and results. If I do provide consent, I may at any time withdraw such consent for specific photographs by contacting **(your business name)**, which will then discontinue the use of said photo(s).

12. _____ I have been given the full opportunity to ask any and all questions which I might have about obtaining semi-permanent cosmetic procedures from a micropigmentation specialist at **(your business name),** and that all of my questions have been answered to my full and total satisfaction.

If you have previously had micropigmentation performed by **(your business name)**, has your medical history changed since you last filled out **(your business name)** Medical History form?

____YES ____NO

If YES, please specify.

_____

_____

I have read and understand the contents of each statement above. I acknowledge that this is a contract and that I have received no warranties or guarantees with respect to the benefits to be realized from or consequences of the aforementioned procedure(s). I further acknowledge that at the time of signing this consent I am of sound mind and capable of making independent decisions for myself. I hereby release and forever discharge and hold harmless **(your business name)** and its owners, managers, employees and affiliates from any and all claims, damages or legal actions arising from or connected in any way with my micropigmentation, or the procedure and conduct used in my performing my tattoo, to the fullest extent allowed by the law.

Name _____Date _____
(Please print legibly)

Client Signature _____Date _____

Parent or Legal Guardian _____Date_____
(If Client Is Under 18)

Practitioner statement:

I have personally reviewed the above information with my client or the client's representative.

Practitioner Signature _____
Date _____

Pre-Procedure Information

*NO BOTOX FOR AT LEAST 2-3 MONTHS PRIOR TO THE PROCEDURE!

IMPORTANT: Please do not wear White/Light color tops on the day of the procedure. Chewing gum is not allowed during the procedure. No one is allowed in the procedure room except for the client, so all guests must wait in the lobby area or leave until the client is ready to be picked up. Thank You

1. Wear your normal brow makeup on the day of the procedure.

2. No eyebrow tinting or dyeing should be done before or after the procedure.

3. Refrain from Retin A (Retinols) cream at least a week prior to the procedure.

4. Acne skin care should only be applied as a spot treatment if needed but not over the whole face.

5. Avoid tweezing or waxing for at least 1-2 weeks prior to the procedure, if possible.

6. Avoid tanning or long exposure to the sun 2 weeks prior to the procedure.

7. Avoid Chemical peels, ablative laser treatment at least a month prior to the procedure.

8. If you had permanent makeup laser removal, must wait 4 weeks before the new application.

9. Remove contact lenses before the procedure, some pressure might be applied to the surrounding of the eye area and could cause discomfort.

10. This procedure can NOT be performed on lactating women; must wait at least 3-6 months after stopping before being considered a candidate for the procedure.

11. Refrain from the use of <u>alcohol</u>, <u>Aspirin</u>, <u>Ibuprofen</u>, <u>Vit-E</u>, <u>Fish Oil</u>, <u>St. John Wort</u>, or any **blood thinners for 7 days before your procedure**. Refrain from judgment-altering drugs for at least 24 hours prior to your procedure. **DO NOT STOP ANY DOCTOR'S PRESCRIPTION/MEDICATION BEFORE CONSULTING YOUR PHYSICIAN FIRST.**

12. A patch test is recommended if you have multiple unknown allergies.

13. If you are diabetic or under serious physician care, consult with your physician regarding this procedure prior to treatment. <u>Written approval from your physician will be required at the time of the procedure.</u>

14. Expect extra sensitivity if you are close, on or right after your monthly menstrual period. If you have a headache, body injury, body ache, stress or lacking sleep. Use Tylenol if needed.

15. Make sure you had a good meal before the procedure. On average, the procedure is 3 ½ hours long and hunger could add to the sensitivity.

16. Avoid exercising at least 3 hours prior to your appointment.

Every individual has their own unique skin; therefore, everyone heals differently and at a different speed. It is important to not schedule any major events for 3 weeks after the initial procedure.

AFTERCARE INSTRUCTIONS

Successful healed result depends on your aftercare. Please follow the instructions below very carefully! Like any cosmetic procedure, it is a process. Please be patient; the healing process takes a few weeks before you can appreciate the result. The healing process is at least 2-3 weeks.

- Do not touch your eyebrows during the whole healing process!

- Do not pick, peel, rub or scratch the micro pigments on the eyebrow. It may cause scarring or loss of pigments.

- Avoid full showers, showering just from the neck down within the first 48 hours.

- After the first 48 hours, clean them gently 1-2 times per day (as instructed) with warm water and baby shampoo using a cotton pad. Movement should be done in the direction of hair growth without forcing the skin (as if you're dusting the skin).

- First 2 mornings, apply a VERY thin layer of the ointment/cream provided using Q-tips (no double dipping, to prevent contamination). Use as directed by your technician. (**Over-applying the ointment can result in pigment loss**). If you have oily or combination skin, dry healing method is more suited for your skin type.

- **Do not** apply A&D ointment, Oils or any antibiotic cream to the area.

- *If you have oily or combination skin type, you will be advised to start cleansing your brows starting the next morning of the procedure. 1-3 times a day based on your activity level for that day. Also, you would need to use oil-absorbent dapping paper throughout the day as many times as possible for the first 3 weeks at least to remove excess oil from your brows and the surrounding areas. NO aftercare ointment/cream would be needed or used.

- There may be some pigment on the cotton pad or Q-tips as you are cleaning or applying the ointment/cream; do not be alarmed! This is just excess pigment and body fluid naturally exiting through the upper layer of the skin. Hair loss is not possible as the blade does not even penetrate deep enough into the skin to reach your hair bulb. On rare occasions, you might notice few actual hair strands as you clean but those are the ones that were already about to fall out anyway.

- Short-term/ long-term care: when applying your skincare, always leave a one-inch gap between your application and your brows; product does migrate and will still reach the area you did not cover. Moisturizers may blur the pigment over time, retinols and Vit C and any exfoliant/brightener ingredients in your skincare could result in premature fading or color discoloration.

  ✓ Next 7 days: fitness and any activities that require effort and sweat are not recommended

  ✓ Next 3 weeks: sauna, Jacuzzi is not allowed.

  ✓ Next 3 weeks: swimming is not allowed. Chlorine can cause irritation to the eyebrow.

  ✓ Next 1-2 weeks: Strictly prohibited from applying foundation or powder **onto** the eyebrow area.

  ✓ Next 1 week: Strictly forbidden sleeping on your stomach where you are face down onto the pillow, or too much on your sides that part of your face is on the pillow. When the pillow is in contact with the eyebrows during healing process, it can rub off some of the pigments in certain areas, causing asymmetrical looks, not to mention you could risk an infection. A Satin pillow case is recommended if you can't control sleeping on your back.

✓ Next 1 month: Strictly prohibited direct exposure to sunlight or any other form of UV rays (tanning, beach). Use hats or visors to protect them and sunscreen if around the pool.

✓ Short-term/long-term aftercare: no abrasive creams, sea salt, or **chemical peels** close or on the brow area. Please advise your aesthetician to apply a line of Aquaphor 5mm above your brow line to avoid migration of the peel into your brows. When getting any laser treatment done to your face, advise the technician to protect the pigment by covering the brows with gauze when getting close to that area.

✓ Other activities you may need to avoid during the first week of the healing process: Performing heavy cleaning tasks of the household where there is a lot of airborne debris. Smoking and alcohol may lead to slow healing.

✓ Next 1 week: If you have pets, avoid getting them too close to your brows.

• All semi-permanent makeup procedures are multi-session processes. You are required to come back for a perfect visit before it can be determined that the work is complete. This visit is scheduled about 6-8 weeks after the initial procedure. Be prepared for the color intensity of your procedure to be significantly sharper, brighter, warmer or darker in the first week than what is expected in the final healed result. It will take time for this transition based on how quickly the outer layer of your skin exfoliates and heals.

- While these injected tones may initially simulate the exact color and tone desired, they will not always remain a perfect match. Injected tones are constant, while our own skin tones will vary depending on exposure to cold, heat, sun and circulatory changes. Since delicate skin or sensitive areas may swell slightly or redden, some clients feel it best not to make social plans for a day or two following their procedure.

- As was explained during the consultation, an initial conservative approach to the application is important until your skin's unique way of healing and retention is determined when you come back for your initial touch-up, easier to add than to reverse the application, therefore, based on your healed result a change to the color (darker), thickness or stroke depth can be applied.

HAPPY HEALING!

Stages of Eyebrow Microblading

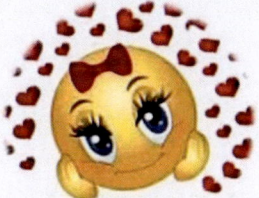

Day 1: OMG! I'm in love with
my new brows. Thank you!

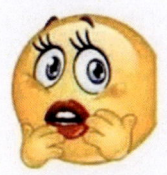

Days 2-4: I don't like this color.
It's too dark.

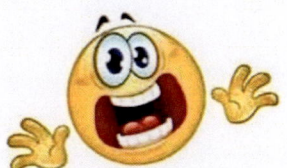

Days 5-7: Oh, no! My brows are
scabbing and falling off.

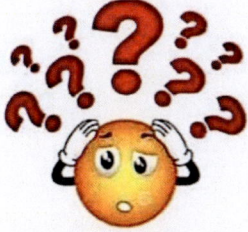

Days 8-10: *?!?!?* My brows
are gone.

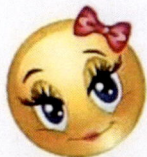

Days 14-28: Thank God my brows
are coming back! Still looking
patchy and uneven.

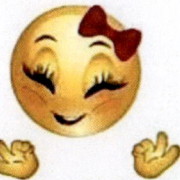

Day 42 (after touch up): Aww, they're
beautiful! I love them! Thanks again!

CORRECTION FORM

CONSENT FORM/DISCLAIMER TO CORRECT PREVIOUSLY MISAPPLIED PERMANENT MAKEUP.

State the procedure(s) that are to be corrected:

_____

Previously applied by: _____.

Date applied _____

State in detail the problem:

_____
_____
_____
_____
_____
_____

I understand that correcting or touching up micropigmentation that was performed by others involves additional risks because of the existence of permanent pigments of unknown composition, brand, color, age, shape and other factors over which (your business name) and its employee has no control. I understand that additional appointments after the initial and follow-up appointments may be required and will be billed at (your business name) standard rates. I understand that (your business name) cannot predict the results in advance and cannot guarantee and has not represented that the results will be as I desire. I understand and fully accept the risks associated with this procedure and hold (your business name) harmless from same.

SIGNATURE: _____Date _____

THE CLIENT STATED THAT HE/SHE HAS READ, UNDERSTOOD AND AGREES WITH THE ABOVE. HE/SHE HAS HAD THE OPPORTUNITY TO ASK ANY QYESTIONS.

TECHNITION: _____Date _____

TOOL CONSENT FORM

I _____ confirm that I checked the manual tools and needles/blades which about to be used by (**your business name**) for my procedure today are fully sealed in their original manufacture seal, indicating and confirming the sanitization of these disposable tools directly from the company.

Signature _____Date _____

Practitioner _____Date _____

Signature _____

CLIENT CHART NOTES

Client: _____ Technician: _____

Consultation Date:

_____

Procedure: _____

Date: _____

Fees Paid: _____

Needle: _____

Color/Mod:

_____

Pic: ____

Procedure: _____

Date: _____

Fees Paid: _____

Needle: _____

Color/Mod: _____

Pic: ____

Procedure: _____

Date: _____

Fees Paid: _____

Needle: _____

Color/Mod: _____

Pic: ____

Procedure: _____

Date: _____

Fees Paid: _____

Needle: _____

Color/Mod: _____

Pic: ____

Procedure Notes:

_____

_____

_____

_____

_____

_____

Chapter 12

SANITATION

&

STERILIZATION

OSHA Requirements. Bloodborne Pathogens

WHAT IS OSHA?

OSHA stands for Occupational Safety and Health Administration. It is a federal agency within the United States Department of Labor. OSHA was established to ensure safe and healthy working conditions for employees in the United States, including sterilization requirements. The agency's primary mission is to set and enforce safety and health standards in the workplace, as well as provide education, training, and assistance to employers and workers.

OSHA developed the Bloodborne Pathogens Standard which is now recognized worldwide. This standard is designed to protect workers from the risk of exposure to Bloodborne Pathogens, such as the Human Immunodeficiency Virus (HIV) and the Hepatitis B and C Virus (HBV)(HCV). The standard was revised by the Needle-stick Safety and Prevention Act of 2000 to set a greater detail and made more specific OSHA's requirement for employers to identify, evaluate and implement safer medical devices.

Note that OSHA standards are federal regulations that apply nationwide, and states can have their own additional regulations or guidelines. Also, keep in mind that regulations can change over time, so it's crucial to check with the most current and authoritative sources.

OSHA's universal requirement and precautions have been broken down into 10 categories, which you will learn about in the Bloodborne Pathogen online training.

- Hand hygiene

- Universal precautions

- Immunizations

- Cleaning and disinfection

- Personal protective equipment PPE

- Safe needle handling practices

- Biohazard labeling requirements

- Waste disposal and linen management

- Exposure control plan

- Post exposure follow up

AWARENESS:

There is always a potential risk of exposure to bloodborne pathogens diseases when doing a PMU procedure. The best way to protect yourself from those risks is by following the universal precautions, meaning that you should always assume that all human blood and body fluids are infectious; you also need to keep in mind that you do not have to see blood or bodily fluids on instruments for an infection to occur.

Bloodborne pathogens are viruses and bacteria carried in the blood and body fluids. It is crucial to be aware of what these pathogens are and how they are transmitted, and most importantly, how to protect yourself from them during a PMU procedure. There are many bloodborne pathogens, including malaria, syphilis, but the most notably;

- HIV/AIDS

- Hepatitis B

- Hepatitis C

(Hepatitis B and C are liver diseases that are fatal)

These diseases can be transmitted through direct or indirect contact like:

- A puncture wound from contaminated sharp objects like a needle, broken glass or all kinds of sharp objects.

- Through mucus membranes such as mouth, eyes or nose.

- Through non-intact skin like sores, rashes, cuts.

PPE GEAR

(Personal Protective Equipment) is a very important step in order to keep potentially infectious fluids off you and your clothes in order to prevent cross contamination protecting yourself and your client. They are;

- Gloves

- Face mask

- Eyewear

- Aprons/Gown

How to practice universal precautions, sanitation, and sterilization, before, during and after in relation to PMU procedures.

These steps are crucial to ensure safety and by diligently following these required precautions, you can help minimize the risk of infection and maintain a professional/ethical practice.

- Use a good daily personal hygiene practice. This includes washing your hands thoroughly with anti-microbial soap and warm water, wearing 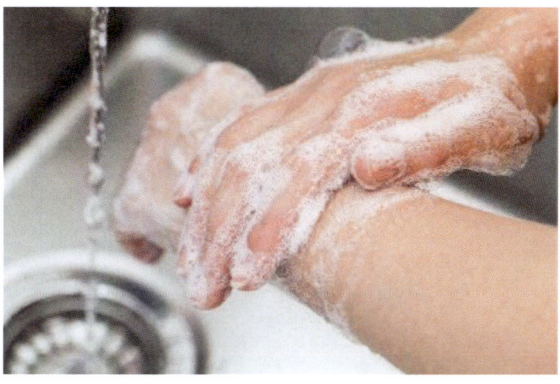 clean appropriate clothing (scrubs).

- Keep your disinfected, sterilized or single-use tools in a properly sealed or closed containers to ensure a sterile environment until ready to be used.

- Make sure you have properly cleaned and organized the workspace prior to the procedure. Wearing gloves, start with disinfecting all surfaces and equipment that will come into contact with the client, including treatment tables, chairs, and trays.

- Use a disposable single-use barrier film or covers to the already disinfected areas of work to prevent contamination of surface. They should be discarded after each client. Wash hands and wear gloves before you touch the already disinfected areas and before organizing your tray with all products, pigment, blade, and all the tools to be used for the procedure.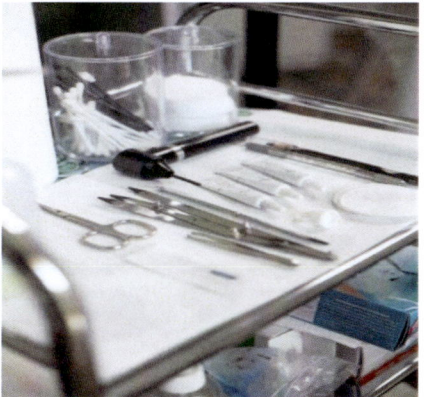

- Wear your PPE gear, new gloves, mask and apron before starting the procedure.

- Change gloves throughout the procedure or as necessary, especially if they become contaminated or torn. Do not touch random surfaces with your contaminated or even non-contaminated gloves (cell phone, cabinet, etc); take off your gloves first and once you are ready to get back to the application, put on new gloves. When removing gloves, turn the glove inside out to contain any contaminants; you can do so by gripping the outer surface of one glove near the cuff and peel it down, remove the second glove by inserting your fingers inside the other cuff and pull it down. Reusable aprons should be placed in designated containers to be washed and decontaminated or even discarded.

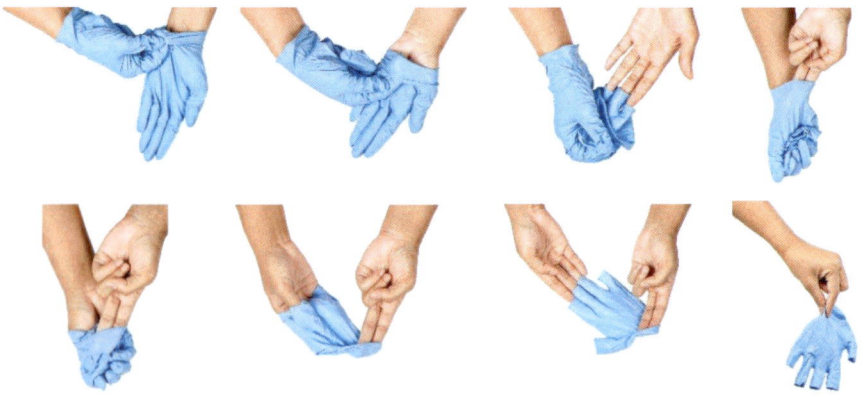

- Your client's skin needs to be cleaned and sanitized with antiseptic solution or 70% alcohol as a first step to starting the procedure.

- Best to remove your contaminated protective equipment with gloves and wash your hands after.

- Contaminated clothes should be washed immediately and separately.

- Setting up and tearing down steps to your work area are equally important to avoid cross-contamination. Never start your clean-up, disinfecting or sterilization process without your protective gear, most importantly your gloves. Start with:

  1. Remove the blade; use a cotton pad to carefully hold the contaminated blade from the lower side part of the blade as you remove it off the hand-held tool. Make sure to twist and loosen up the grip for an easier removal.

  2. Place reusable tools in the sink for proper cleaning before disinfecting and/or sterilization. Wash thoroughly with anti-microbial soap using a metal bristle brush, rinse well, then immerse your reusable tools (handheld tool, tweezers and seizors) in BARBICIDE pre-mixed solution for an average of 20 minutes. Other reusable items that cannot be immersed in the liquid can be sprayed or wiped thoroughly with BARBICIDE wipes, like (digital measuring tools, pigment bottles, numbing bottles, calipers, markers, and so on)

  3. Discard all wastes and single-use tools generated during the procedure (swabs, cotton pads, etc); anything that has been contaminated with blood and body fluid should be disposed of in designated biohazard container or bag to be picked up by a bio-hazard waste company.

  4. Disinfect all the surfaces (table, ring light, chair and so on) of the area of work with BARBICIDE wipes, or can be sprayed with BARBICIDE for 10 minutes and wiped off thereafter.

5. Back to the immersed tools, use a tong to collect out the tools for a complete rinse; if you are using a BARBICIDE jar, easier to lift the metal basket inside and use glovers to pick up the tools for a thorough rinse. Fully dry the tools and have them packaged for autoclave sterilization; follow the specific and instructed time and heat measurement requirement by the manufacturer for your unit. Also, packages should contain an integrator or process indicator. After the sterilization, if a sterile pack is compromised, the tool shall be re-sterilized again before use.

6. Disinfect your sink with BARBICIDE wipe or spray.

7. Maintain detailed records of your sanitation and sterilization process, including dates, methods, and equipment used; this documentation can be important for regulatory compliance in some states, <u>that's why it is very important to contact your state's Health Department to be well-informed and aware of your state requirement and regulation since it varies from one state to another.</u>

TOOLS CATEGORY

- **Disposable single-use includes:**
  - ➢ Individually wrapped and sealed blades/needles
  - ➢ One-unit single-use microblading manual tool
  - ➢ Pigment plastic rings and cups
  - ➢ Eyebrow razors

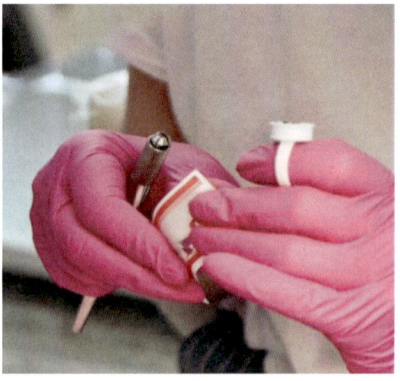

- ➢ Cotton tip swabs
- ➢ Micro brushes or brow brushes
- ➢ Flocked applicators
- ➢ Cotton pads or gauze
- ➢ Gloves
- ➢ Protecting film or cover
- ➢ Measuring ruler stickers
- ➢ Drape sheets
- ➢ Masks

- **Disinfected reusable tools include: Method of disinfection (BARBICIDE liquid immersion and BARBICIDE wipe)**
  - ➢ Pigment bottles/containers
  - ➢ Calipers

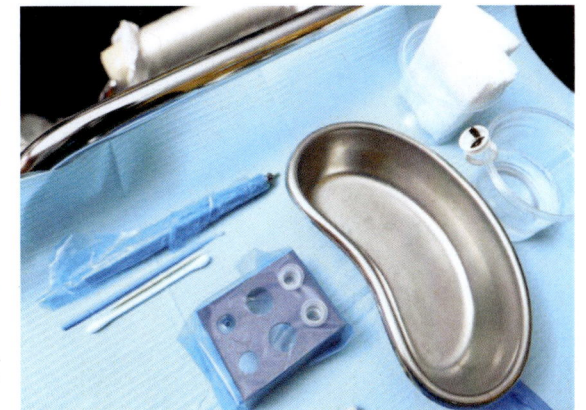

  - ➢ Pencils and markers
  - ➢ Power supplies (ring light as example)
  - ➢ Pigment or numbing cup holders
  - ➢ Machine or manual tool holder, if applicable
  - ➢ Kidney or medical trays
  - ➢ Magnifying glasses, if applicable

➢ Numbing bottle solution

- **Sterilized reusable tools: Method of sterilization (Autoclave)**

  ➢ Reusable metal

  ➢ microblading manual hand-held tool

  ➢ Tweezers

  ➢ Scissors

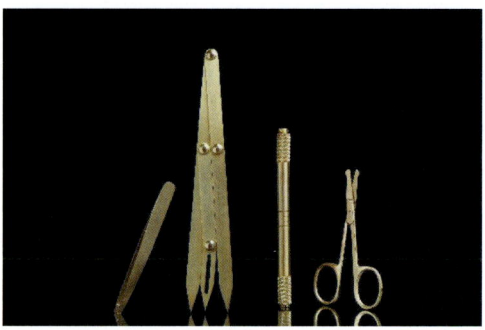

REQUIRED AND MUST-HAVE:

1. Reliable Autoclave unit (use process-only indicator sterilizing packages)

2. BARBICIDE (liquid-wipes) EPA-registered hospital disinfectant kills HIV-1, Hepatitis B, Hepatitis C, and numerous other pathogens. Germicidal, fungicidal, and virucidal. Complies with OSHA's Bloodborne Pathogen standard. Pleasant fragrance. Safe for acrylic tanning beds, stainless steel, plastics, combs, brushes, rollers, and shears.

3. Reliable PPE gear (gloves, masks, apron/gown)

4. Sharps container

5. Blood Spill Kit

6. HBV immunization

7. Bloodborne pathogens certification

8. Certification or license

9. Proper workspace

   - Clean facility

- Adequate lighting

- Proper ventilation

- Sink with hot and cold running water

- Preferably a touchless soap dispenser and towels

- Proper and clean toilets

- Washable and smooth non-absorbent surfaces, including walls, floors, and furniture

Furthermore:

1. Prior to the procedure, you should obtain a signed informed consent from clients, explaining the risks, benefits, healing and aftercare. Also, explaining that PMU pigments are not FDA-approved and can result in unpredictable health reactions.

2. There is an age restriction for clients receiving permanent makeup services, typically requiring clients to be of a certain age (18 years or older); a parent consent is required if the client is underage.

3. Documentation can help reduce liability and legal risks in the event of a client injury or infection, a good defense against legal claims.

4. Compliance with local regulations, so research and comply with any local, state, or national regulations that pertain to the practice of permanent makeup. These regulations can vary significantly, and some areas may have specific and strict rules that you need to be informed with.

It's important to note that the regulations for permanent makeup can change, and they may vary depending on your location as mentioned above, even within the same state you are conducting your business. Therefore, it's crucial to contact your local Health Department or Cosmetology board if it regulates permanent makeup just to ensure you are in compliance with all applicable rules and requirements.

OSHA has requirements that companies must follow if there is a possibility of employee exposure to bloodborne pathogens in the workplace:

- A written exposure control plan that contains information and procedures to protect employees from exposure and transmission of bloodborne pathogens in the workplace.

- PPE for employees who may come in contact with bloodborne pathogens as part of their work activity.

- Employee training on the risks of exposure and how to protect themselves from exposure.

- Hepatitis B vaccination for any practitioner who may have exposure to bloodborne pathogens.

- Follow-up and evaluation include a written report as well as the appropriate tests and consulting for the employee.

- The source of exposure is also asked to take a blood test and supply the results, but this person has the right to decline the test.

- Confidential medical records must also be kept for all employees with a risk of exposure on the job.

What To Do If You Are Exposed?

If you are exposed to bloodborne pathogens, it is crucial to take immediate and appropriate steps to protect your health and safety. Here are some repeated guidelines and more:

1. Wash the affected area if the exposure involves contact with your skin, mucous membranes, or eyes. Wash the area thoroughly with soap and water, and use plenty of water to rinse and remove any potentially infectious materials.

2. Seek medical evaluation as soon as possible after exposure. Contact a healthcare provider, clinic, or hospital immediately. Make sure to inform the medical personnel about the details of the exposure, including the source of exposure and the nature of the contact.

3. Keep detailed records of the exposure incident. This documentation should include information about the exposure and any actions taken. This is essential for potential follow-up and reporting.

4. Post-Exposure Prophylaxis (PEP), depending on the specifics of the exposure, a healthcare provider may recommend post-exposure prophylaxis, which involves taking antiretroviral medication to reduce the risk of HIV transmission. PEP is most effective when initiated as soon as possible after exposure, so it's important not to delay seeking medical care.

5. Your healthcare provider may recommend testing for bloodborne pathogens (HIV, HBV, and HCV). It is necessary to undergo follow-up testing to ensure that you have not contracted and infection.

6. Depending on your workplace, you are required to report the exposure incident to your employer, as well as to the appropriate occupational health and safety authorities. Be sure to follow your workplace's protocols for reporting incidents.

Remember, preventative measures of proper safety and infection control protocols by using personal protective equipment and getting vaccinated (as in the case of HBV) prevent exposure to bloodborne pathogens, especially in high-risk occupations.

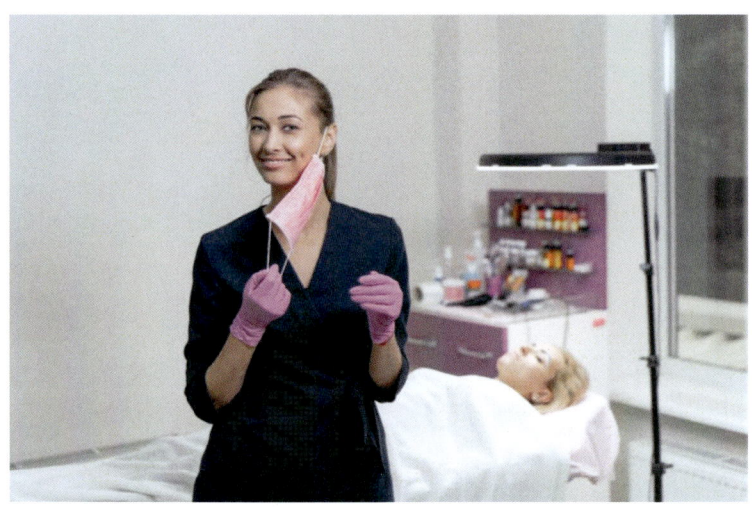

Chapter 13

STROKE PATTERN, DEPTH

&

SKIN STRETCHING

STROKE PATTERN

Stroke patterns refer to the specific way in which individual "hair-like" strokes are drawn, positioned, angled, and connected during the microblading process to create a natural and realistic appearance of the eyebrows. A good stroke pattern should mimic the natural flow and direction of the client's existing brow hairs; this helps achieve a more authentic look. There are numerous stroke patterns created by many artists; some of these patterns may look good on a paper or practice sheets but, in reality, does not always translate well to a natural look when applied to a client; also, the risk of pigment migration is greater due to the close placement of the strokes and the way they are connected. So, rather than rigidly following and adhering strictly to predefined stroke patterns "the cookie cutter approach", it's essential to follow logical and artistic guidelines when performing your strokes. Practice is crucial in perfecting the technique of creating natural looking eyebrows; it helps build the necessary skill and confidence to create customized results for each client.

Different people have different natural hair patterns, same with different ethnicities. Some will have brows where the hair grows naturally downwards, sideways or naturally fluffy. It is ideal to master a universal pattern then alter as needed based on your client's natural brow. Several different strokes can be used throughout the procedure on different part of the eyebrow. First step: practice by drawing your strokes in different directions, curves and shapes so they can flow naturally during the actual application. Second step: once you are confident with drawing single strokes, start practicing combining spine strokes (main strokes) with supporting strokes (shorter strokes) to learn how to merge them together seamlessly. The purpose of patterns is to ensure that you are creating a mirror effect where the right and the left brow are a reflection of each other to achieve a super realistic effect.

Spine strokes start from the base, going upward and run along the initial thickness or half way in of the brow then gradually and diagonally for whatever length chosen throughout the brow towards the tail, so they are longer and are your main guideline for more strokes to be applied. Supporting strokes start midway and merge into the spine strokes; they are shorter in length and can be used to fill in some of the gaps between the main strokes if needed (nanoblading is great for supporting strokes). Strokes should never be drawn parallel to each other, rather in a feathering manner instead. NEVER cut across another stroke as this will lead to blotching of pigment. Make sure to always create a good "void" between strokes to avoid pigment migration; it is very important to do so otherwise, your strokes can merge together.

Here are some examples of universal brow patterns I created for you.

This example is ideal for anyone, especially for brows that naturally grow in different directions. Fluffier fronts, bottom strokes curved diagonally upward and the top pointing downwards. First image showing "spine strokes" only, meaning the main strokes. The next step after applying spine strokes you would be applying "support strokes" as indicated with the yellow color in the second image. Now keep in mind, sometimes and especially with brow that naturally have a good amount of hair, spine strokes alone are good enough.

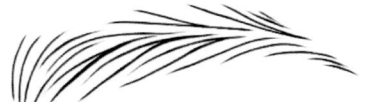 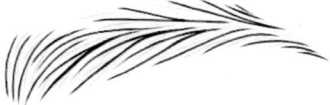

This example is ideal for anyone with brow hairs with a fluffier front, then downwards from the arch point to the tails. (Image created with spine strokes and supporting strokes)

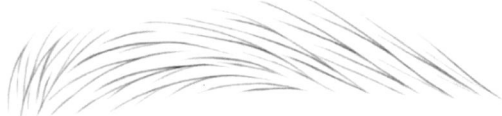

This example is ideal for anyone with fluffy upward brow hair. (Image created with spine strokes and supporting strokes)

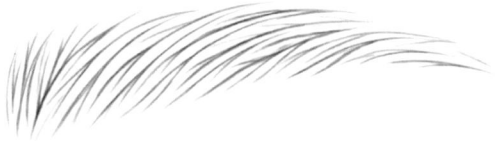

Note: As we learned from previous chapters, some brows hair can be partially non-existing, missing the start of the brow or the tail; when filling in the missing parts, ensure a gradual transition from the natural brow to the created part. Avoid abrupt changes in thickness or shape, as this can make the result look unnatural.

PRESSURE & DEPTH

There are many factors to creating beautiful healed microblading results, like choosing the right pigment, pattern flow and design, but most importantly, the depth of each stroke. So, how deep should your stroke be? This part can be tricky because it all depends on the skin you are working with, how thick or thin their epidermis layer is.

It is crucial to understand this very important part of the application in order to create crisp strokes that won't blur and to be honest, it is what will set the standard for the quality of work you deliver to your clients.

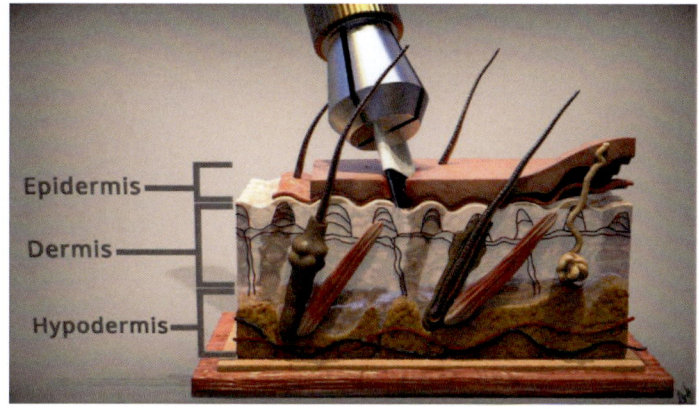

By Sergun Kuyucu

DEPTH

The depth of microblading strokes should be adjusted based on the client's skin. Thickness varies from person to person, so you need to assess the

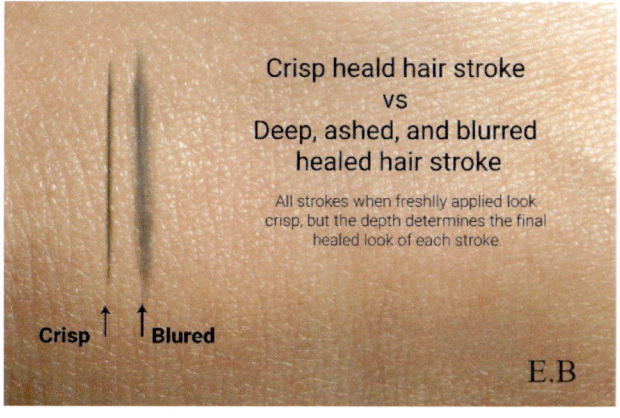

client's skin to determine the appropriate depth. The best approach would be to create your first stroke in the skin with a very light pressure to determine how thick or thin the skin is in order to reach the "sweet spot" (the bottom part of the epidermis above the dermis layer). You will know you are at the right depth when you see very little amount of pinpoint bleeding or when you see a very fine split or sometime when you hear a grating sound. You can go over the same stroke once if need be but no more; it is important to not over do it because if you go too deep (into the layers below the epidermis), you can cause scarring and the color will heal too ashy and dark, on the other hand if you go too shallow, the color won't retain. I'm not going to lie; it is tricky! So, play it safe at first until you get more experienced on how to determine the depth. You can always add more color and depth to your stroke when your client come back for their touch up, especially if your initial stroke was too shallow to retain any pigment. Never panic! Always remember, a completely faded stroke is much easier to fix than a deep ashed out stroke. Important note: the skin is much thinner at the tail of the eyebrow than the start/blub of the brow, so you most definitely need to adjust your pressure when you work on the tail.

ANGLE

Unfortunately, sometimes and especially when you are a new artist, most of the focus goes on how to draw and direct the flow of the stroke while unintentionally not paying attention to the angle of the blade. If you are <u>not</u> penetrating the skin at a perpendicular angle, the quality of the stroke will be compromised and the stroke will be <u>blurry and heal thicker</u>. The blade should be fitted at an angle of 155 degrees into the microblading pen so that by keeping the pen in upright position, all needles are entering into the skin at the same time at a 90-degree angle (upright position). The blade should enter the skin correctly in order to implement pigment successfully, **upright and at <u>a 90-degree angle</u>.**

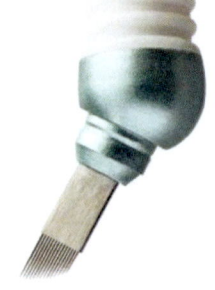

3-POINT STRETCHING

Proper stretch to skin during the application is very important to implement the pigment in a smooth single stroke. Skin is stretched in 3 opposite directions to give the maximum stretch and keep the surface taut and smooth. If you are right-handed, for example, the 2-point stretching would be done with your left hand (the one not holding the tool), pinning the skin down and stretch it apart in small sections; at the same time the pinky of your right hand (holding the tool) must stretch the opposite direction.

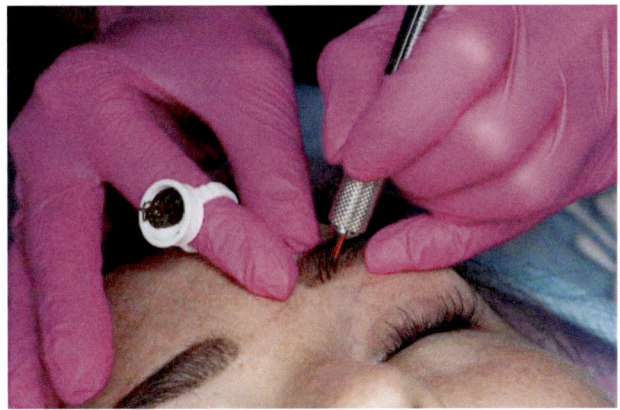

CONSISTENCY

Consistency applies to pressure, speed, steady hand, angle and proper spacing. Maintain a steady hand, and adopt a comfortable posture during the procedure, this ensures stroke control. Work slow to also ensure proper application. Apply a consistent but gentle pressure with the microblading tool, so avoid pressing too hard as it can result in uneven and deep strokes. Remember to keep your angle consistent as well as being consistent with the proper spacing between the strokes, avoid overcrowding or leaving noticeable gaps between strokes.

FOCUS ON ALL FIVE

1. Pressure and Depth

2. Angle

3. 3-point stretch

4. Stroke flow

5. Consistency

The key to success in all five is to practice at all times on different forms. Start with stroke flow on paper first, then start practicing on latex skin to properly draw your strokes with the blade while practicing the angle, and finally, test and practice your depth on fruits like bananas, peaches and oranges. You also can create couple of tiny strokes on yourself to practice the 3-point stretch; most people try it on their thighs. When you are brave enough to draw your first real stroke on your thigh, make sure not to apply any pressure at first; just have the blade glide as if you were holding a feather, next apply a light pigment to the stroke and rub it in and wait couple of minutes for the pigment to absorb, when you clean the area and see the tiny stroke you created, you will realize how easy it is for the blade to cut the skin with the least amount of pressure applied, it will most definitely give you a better understanding to "pressure." All I can tell you is that practicing creates perfection and once you master the application, you can guarantee great results for your clients.

Chapter 14

THE PROCEDURE, STEP BY STEP

THE PROCEDURE, ARE YOU READY?

Nervous? Don't be!

First and foremost, taking slow, deep breaths can help calm your nerves and reduce anxiety; its simple but effective technique to stay composed. Make sure you are well-prepared for the task at hand, review your training, knowledge, and techniques before you begin. Focus on the progress you've made and the hard work you've put into your training. Try to shift your self-talk from self-doubt to self-encouragement, remind yourself of your skills and the positive outcomes you aim to achieve. Start slow and learn from your mistakes. Understand that mistakes can happen, especially when you're still gaining experience. Instead of dwelling on them, view them as opportunities for growth and improvement. Maintain a professional manner and confidence, follow safety protocols to ensure the best possible outcome for your client. After the procedure, take time to reflect on what went well and what could be improved. Remember that continuous learning and self-improvement are essential in any field. Over time, as you gain more experience and become more comfortable with your work, the initial nervousness will diminish. I promise you, it's a natural part of the learning and growth process. You can do this!

Numb Or Not to Numb the Skin?

Different artists with different opinions, it all comes down to what works best for you. Some artists don't believe in numbing agents because they feel it changes the texture of the skin, leaving it soft and soggy which makes it harder to cut through the skin properly. Some artist prefers to work without numbing to save time since numbing can add to the overall duration of the microblading procedure.

However, there are some disadvantages if you don't use numbing. Here's why:

- The increased discomfort experienced by clients during the procedure especially for individuals with low pain tolerance makes the procedure very hard to tolerate; they tense and most likely to bleed more as well. Also, they might include their painful experience in a review, which can potentially harm your business and scare off potential clients.

- Clients may experience more noticeable immediate side effects, such as redness and swelling. These side effects require more time to subside.

- Most importantly, without numbing there is an increased risk of involuntary movements or twitching by clients due to discomfort and these movements can lead to uneven application, resulting in various stroke depth and less desirable as well as less symmetrical brows.

That's why I am a big believer of numbing the skin before and during the application. I advise you to do the same. Remember, quality work is very important!

Let Us Start with the Steps, Shall We?

- Prepare your work space, wear your gloves and thoroughly clean and sanitize all surfaces, equipment, and tools to maintain a sterile and safe environment. Setup your table, get your PPE gear, tools, lights, etc, ready before your client arrive and for easy access during the procedure.

- Do a mini consultation to refresh your client's memory on what was discussed during the initial consultation, especially regarding the desired shape and answer any new questions or concerns she might have. Briefly explain the steps you'll be taking during the procedure; providing a step-by-step overview can help ease your client's nervousness by explaining the process. It also gives them a sense of control and understanding of what's happening.

- Ask your client if there have been any changes in their medical history, medications, or health status since the initial consultation; this is important to assess if any new conditions or medications could impact the procedure. Make sure the consent is signed and dated.

- Show her the blade in its original manufacture seal placed in your tray, and have her sign the tool form.

- Take photos, 5 different angles, from one side of the face to the other side.

- Put your PPE gear on as you will start direct physical contact with the pre-sanitized/sterilized tools and surfaces at this point. Change your gloves often throughout the procedure.

- Have your client lay down, cleanse and sanitize her brow and forehead area.

- Start with measuring and mapping the brows, and follow step by step:

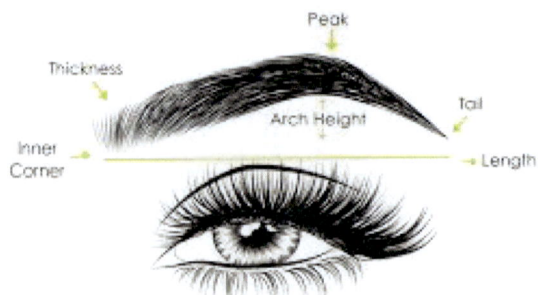

Start by measuring the distance between the eyes at the Tear-duct point , say its roughly about 3 cm, create a center dot at 1-1/2 cm, draw an upward line from this center point to create your middle line (center of the nose)

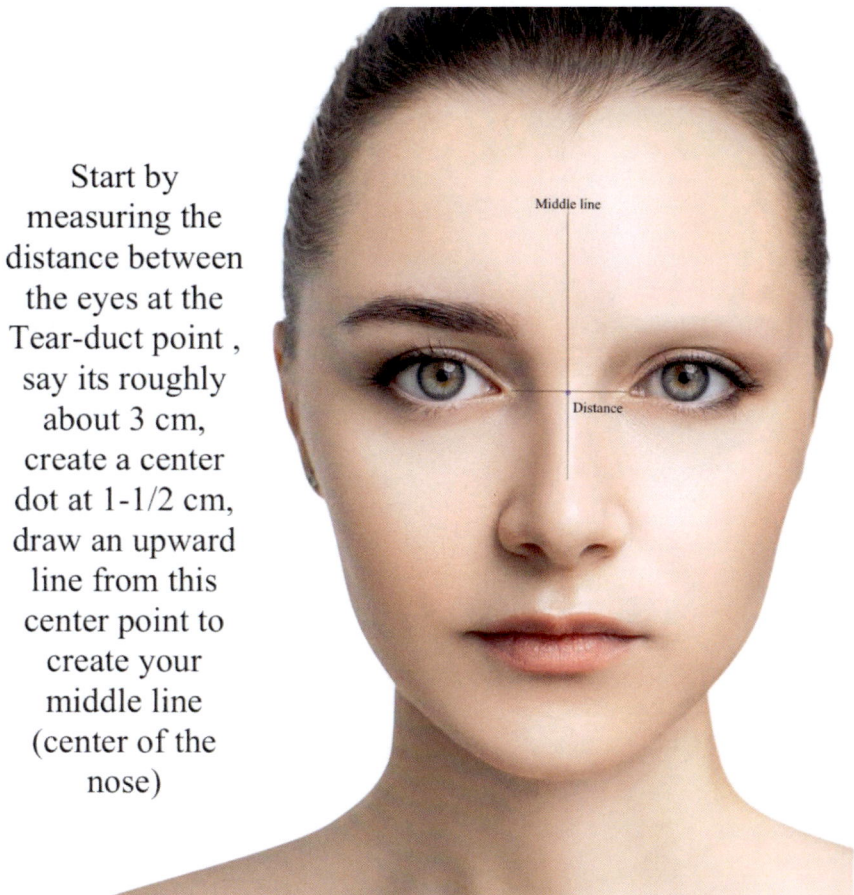

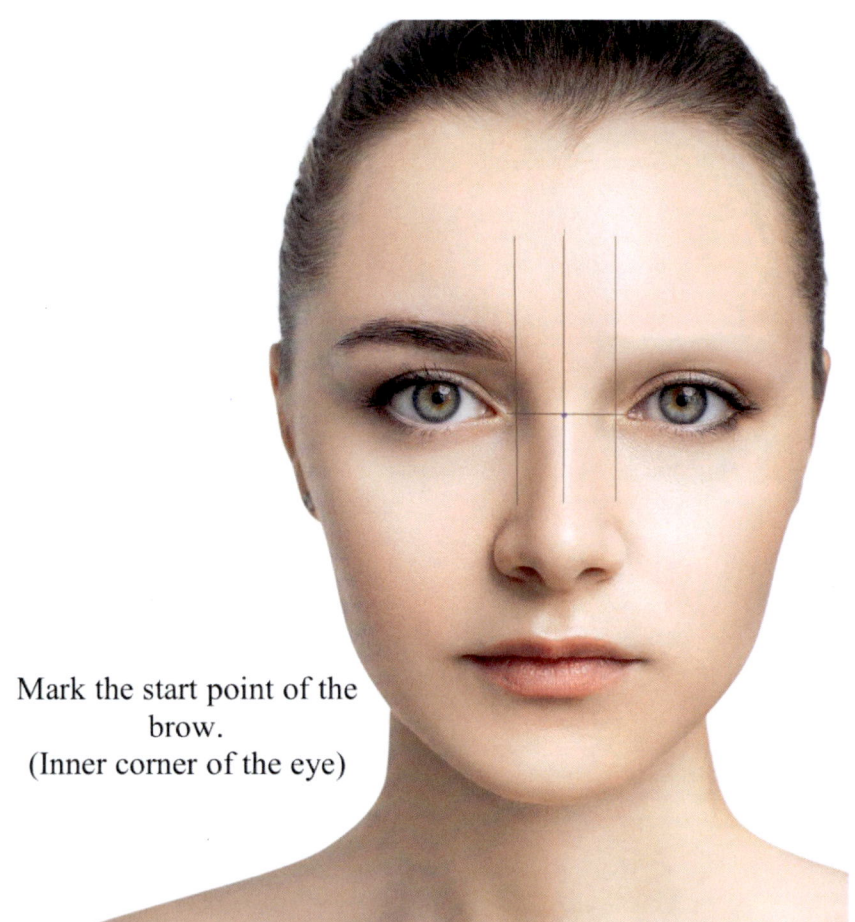

Mark the start point of the
brow.
(Inner corner of the eye)

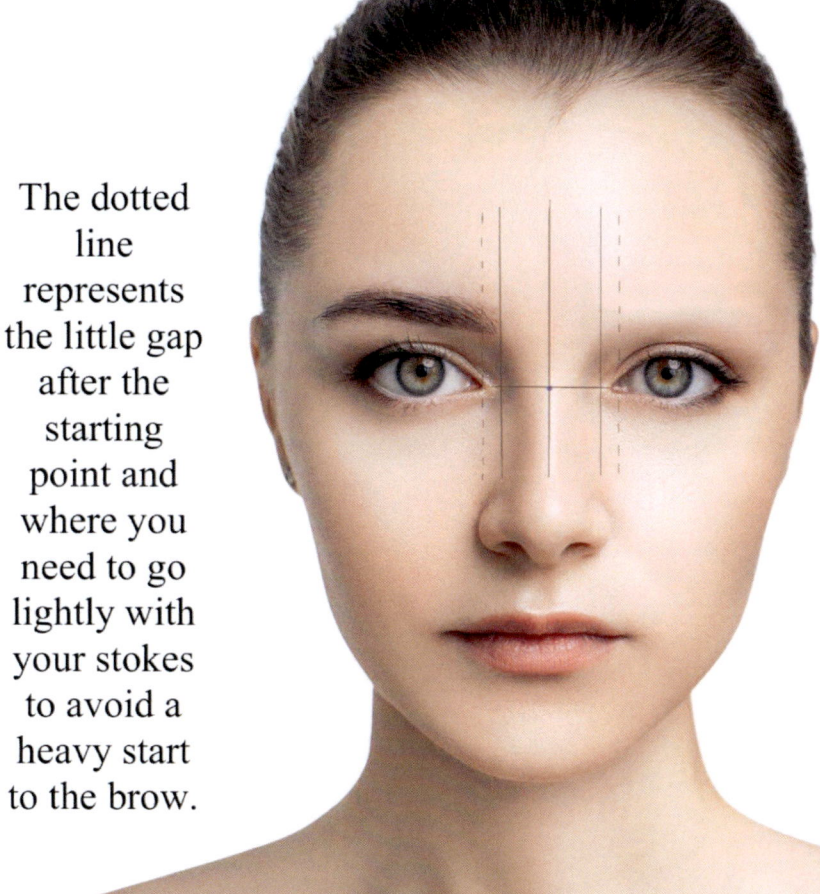

The dotted line represents the little gap after the starting point and where you need to go lightly with your stokes to avoid a heavy start to the brow.

The dotted line can also represent different starting points based on the distance between the eyes. For close set eyes go with the dark dotted line starting at tear ducts. For far set eyes, go with the pink dotted line starting on the inner bridge of the nose.

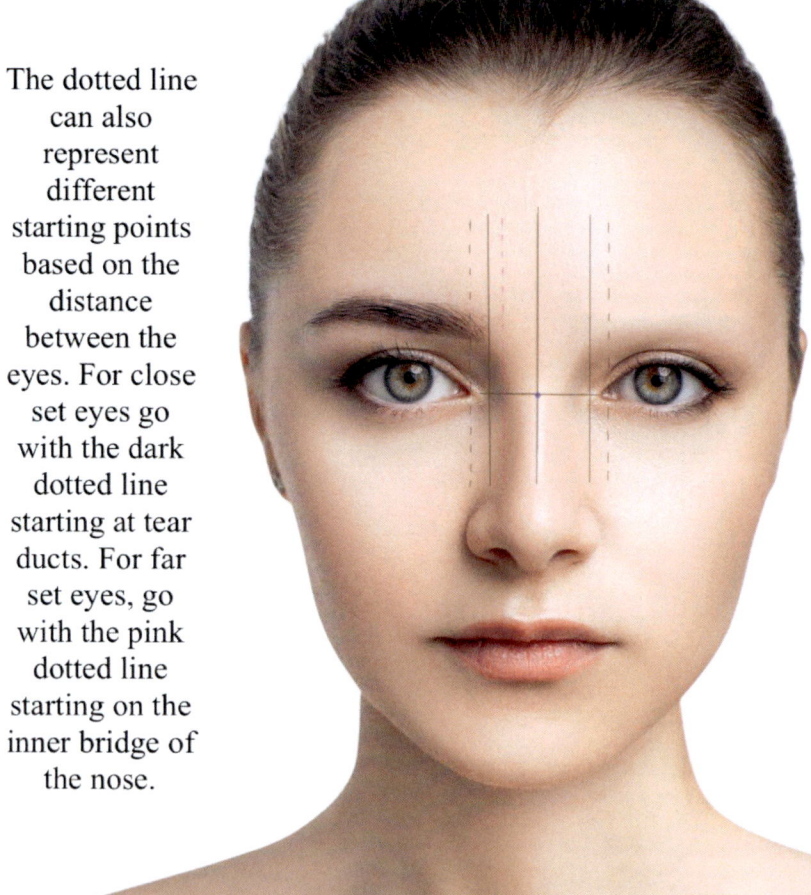

Mark the arch point in 3 ways:

1- Cupid's bow, diagonal line over the pupil.

2- Use the measured distance between the eyes.

3- Mark the tail point first, divide the length of the brow into three sections, the 2/3 is your mark.

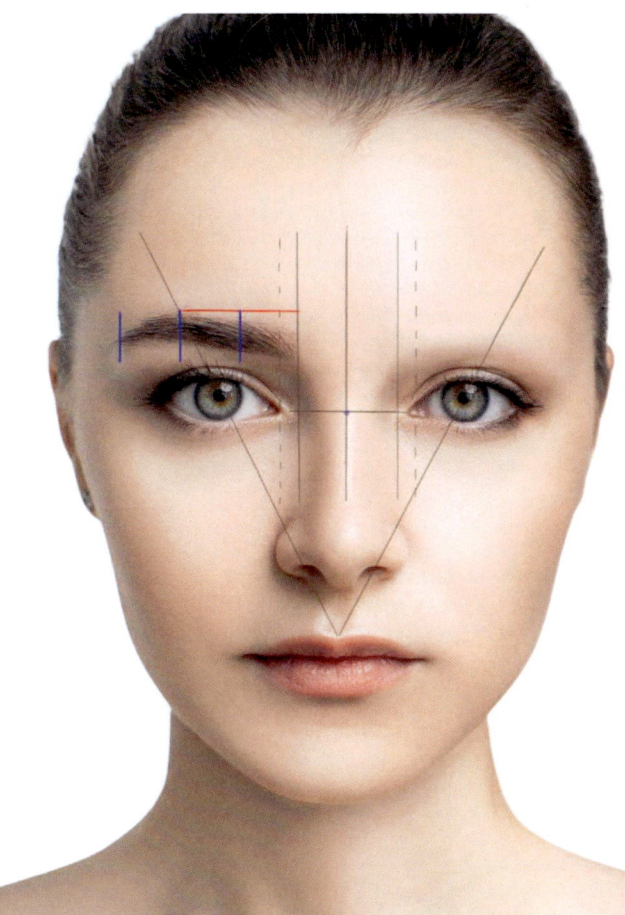

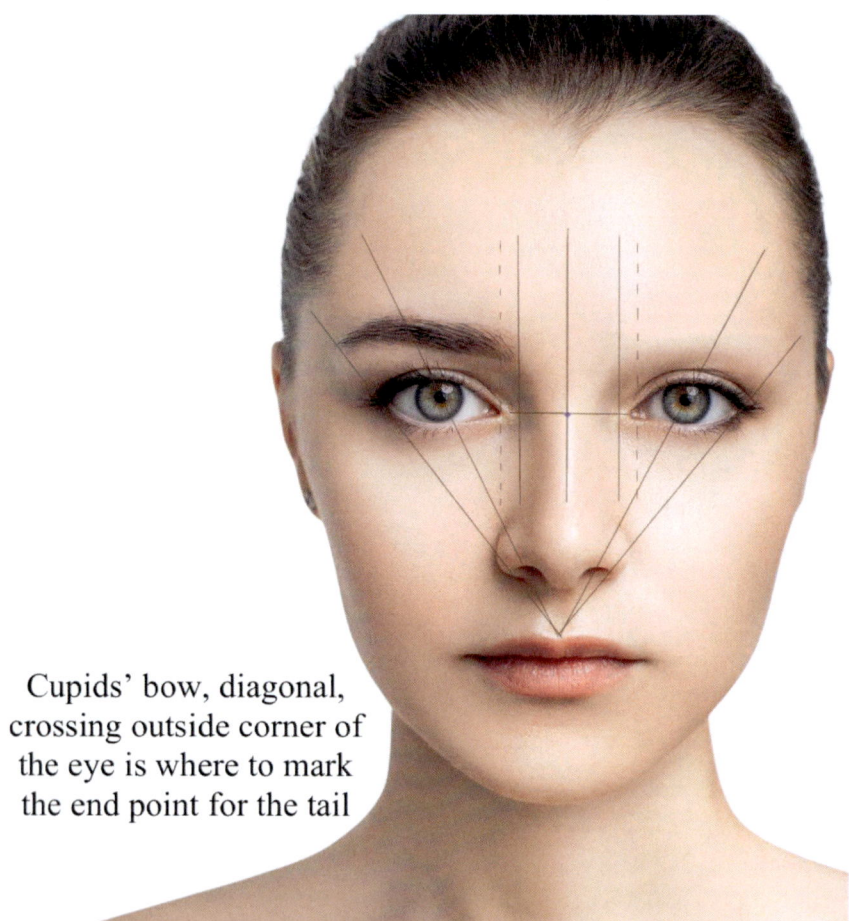

Cupids' bow, diagonal,
crossing outside corner of
the eye is where to mark
the end point for the tail

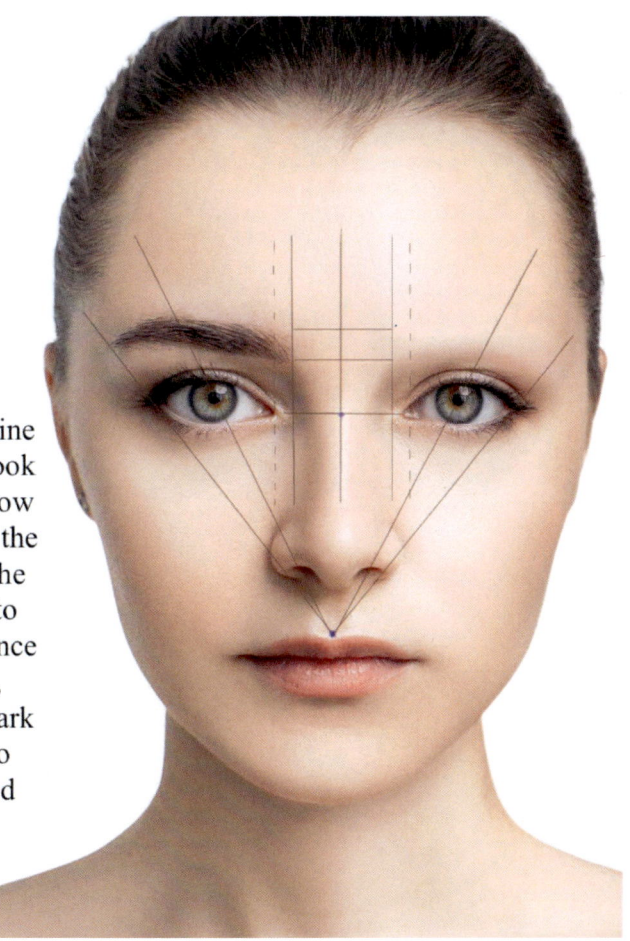

Front point baseline and thickness. Look for the curved brow bone right above the eye socket and the closest section to the start point. Once you marked it, create another mark right above it to mark the desired thickness.

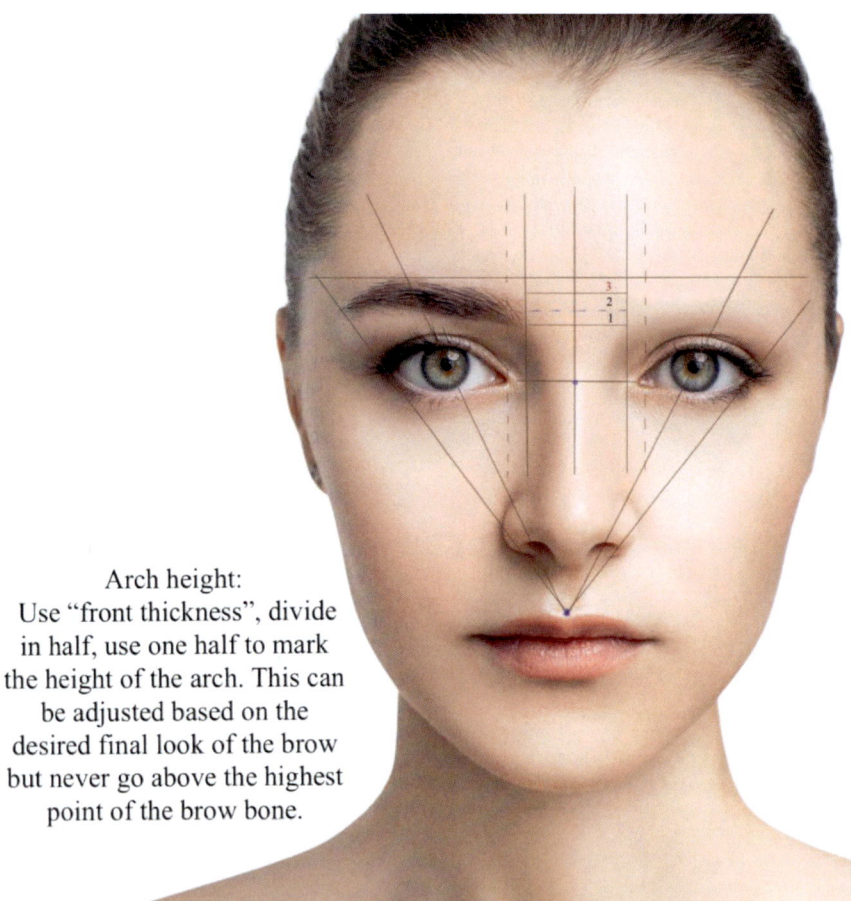

Arch height:
Use "front thickness", divide
in half, use one half to mark
the height of the arch. This can
be adjusted based on the
desired final look of the brow
but never go above the highest
point of the brow bone.

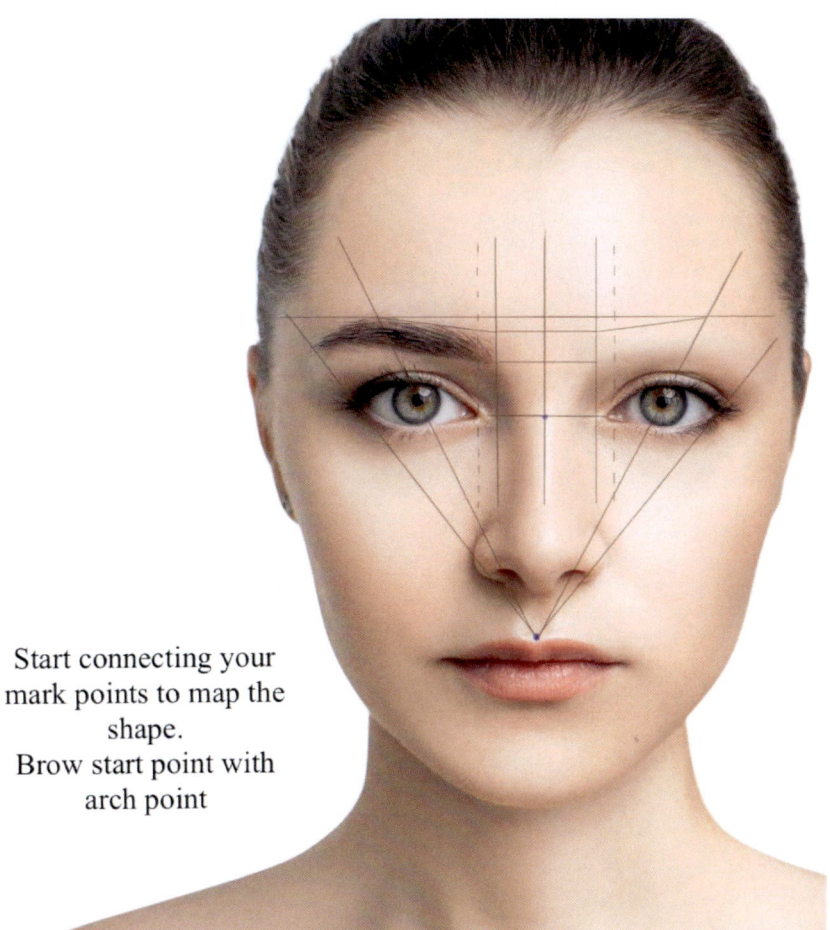

Start connecting your mark points to map the shape.
Brow start point with arch point

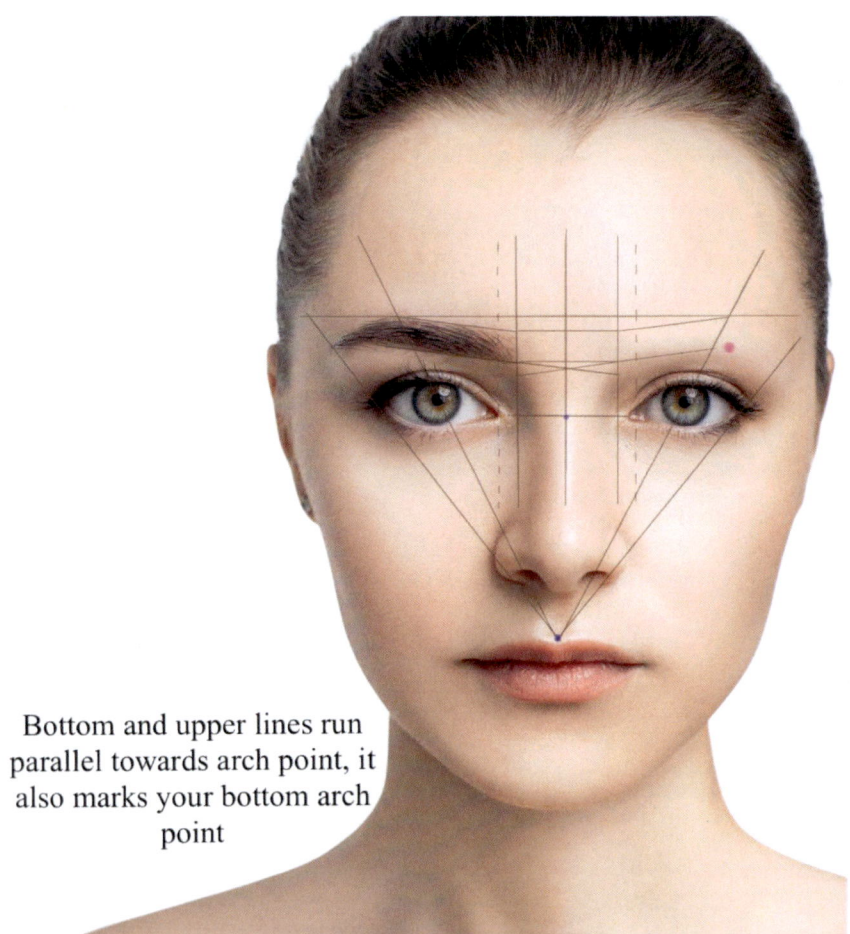

Bottom and upper lines run parallel towards arch point, it also marks your bottom arch point

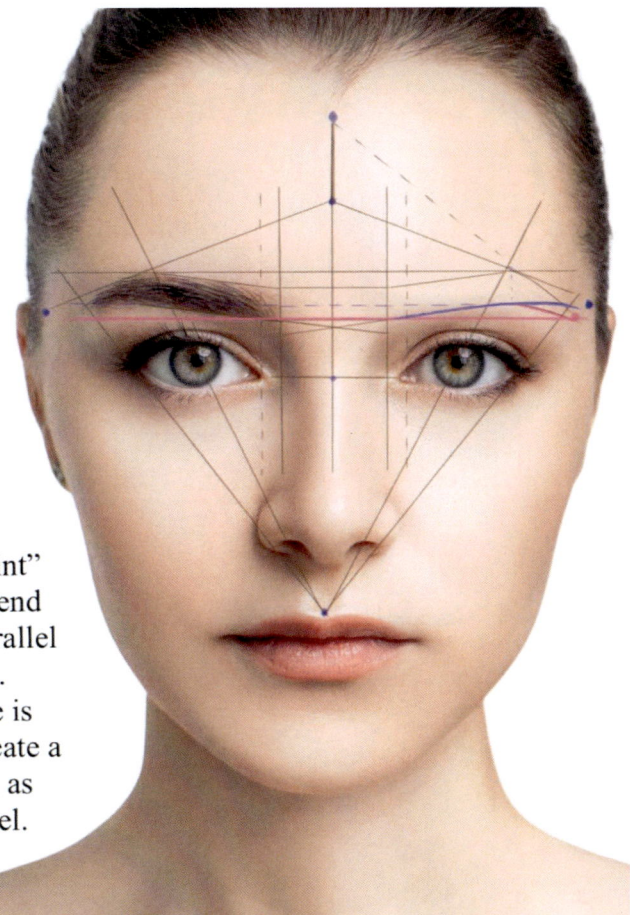

Connect arch point with tail end.

Bottom of "start point" and bottom of "tail end point" should run parallel as shown in pink. The blue doted line is when you want to create a slightly higher tail, as shown on the model.

- Now that you have mapped the brows, remove all the measurement lines you created, leaving only the outline of the design, otherwise your client will be very confused.

- Ask your client to sit up at this point and hand her the mirror to check your design; ask her if she wants anything to be adjusted to her desire (thinner, thicker, higher arch) and if you find fit then go ahead and make the adjustment, if you don't believe it's the right move then explain your concern of her request. This is a very important step; it is your final approval from your client regarding the shape.

- Next step is color matching; you want to choose the closest pigment color to her natural brow hair. Remember, in order to create the most natural outcome, you would need to make it look like she just grew a bunch of her own natural hair back, meaning the color, stroke size and stroke flow need to flow perfectly with her existing natural brow. As you know by now, brown comes in different shades and base tones (warm/cool/neutral) and (light/dark). Choose few pigments and apply small amount of these colors individually on her forehead to mix with her natural lipids and allow them to oxidize.

- Pre-numb the brows with 5% lidocaine numbing cream for 20-30 min.

- Next, remove the cream by dapping it off gently without messing your drawn design; hand her the mirror to be a part of matching the pigment with her natural color; at this point, you are able to see which pigment is pulling warm or cool on her skin and it will give you an overall idea which color is most suited to her natural brow color and skin tone. Don't drag this step too long; you don't want the numbing to wear off before you start.

- At this point and fairly quick, you can go over the outlined design again with a white marker or white paste to help keeping your original lines crisp and free form smudging. You can also pre draw your main strokes at this point if you want or at least section the brow to 3 sections to help you direct the angle of strokes applied.

- Directly or indirectly have your client witnessed you opening the new and sterilized blade pouch and place it inside the manual tool.

- Apply your main strokes to lock in the shape; don't overfill the brow at this point. Leave room for adjustment if needed.

- Clean the brows with (baby shampoo/water) mixture to remove the pigment that has been mixed with pinpoint bleeding and any lymph fluids; dry, then apply a fresh layer of pigment over the brow to absorb properly for about 10 min. This is very important especially with older, thin skin, because they are prone to bleeding more than the average, the mixture of old blood and pigment will heal gray or black and it's very difficult to correct.

- After the 10 minutes period, clean the brows and apply a secondary numbing gel to diffuse the redness and pain since they will be feeling sore at this point. Take advantage of these 5 min to go over the aftercare with your client in details.

- Remove the gel and hand her the mirror to have a look; at this point she is finally seeing what you have been working on right from the start. A lot of times, clients are satisfied with only one pass of strokes, especially when they see their brows looking fluffy and natural; however, some clients will want more definition; this is when you start with your second pass, filling slightly more in between the main strokes. Remember, you must leave negative space between strokes to keep them looking soft and natural, but most importantly to avoid pigment migration, especially on oily skin.

- Once the application is complete and the skin has been numbed with a secondary numbing gel defusing the redness and any irritation, you can start with the after-photos, following the same angles as you did initially. It is important to show your client her B&A photos before she leaves and even send her a copy if she requests.

- Make sure to schedule her touch-up appointment and hand her the aftercare hydrating product before she leaves.

Chapter 15

AFTERCARE, HEALING STAGES

&

TOUCH-UPS

Aftercare

This is the part where you sadly not in control! All you can hope for is for your client to take the aftercare instructions seriously and follow them diligently to avoid and minimize the risk of complication and ensure the best results. First and foremost, your client needs to understand that everyone's skin heals differently, so the timeline for the healing process may vary and their skin type can play a big factor on the healing part and retention. Furthermore, there are two parts to the aftercare, short-term care and long-term care so they need to understand that it is solely on them to make sure their beautiful brows don't discolor or prematurely fade due to their daily habits and lifestyle. Initially, clients are excited and loving their brows, but overtime, they unfortunately forget how important to still care for them that's why you need to know that the sun, chlorine water and skincare products are every artist's nightmare!

Remind your client that:

- Microblading is a semi-permanent cosmetic procedure; following the aftercare properly can significantly affect how long the results last.

- The procedure involves making small incisions in the skin and depositing pigment, basically creating small, superficial wounds which require proper hygiene and aftercare to support the healing and recovery process. Failing to do so can lead to complications, slower healing, and infections.

- Proper care and using the hydrating cream minimize discomfort due to itching or any possible irritation during the healing process. It also minimizes excessive scabbing, pigment loss or uneven healing.

- Long-term care is just as important as short-term care, often exposures to external factors like the sun, pools (chorine water), and skincare products can be too harsh and cause the pigment to fade prematurely. Obviously, you cannot stop them from living their life but make it your responsibility to at least educate them on how to protect their brow while living their normal lifestyle. It is better to wear a hat instead of sunscreen (a lot of sunscreens are tinted and have moisturizer), but if this option is not available or the client is hanging by the pool, she would require sunscreen and if she desire to be inside the pool then it is best to cover the brow with a thin layer of Aquaphor as a barrier.

- When applying skincare products, tell them to leave an inch above the brow free from product application, product migrate and that area will still get covered eventually but at least the product won't reach the pigment. Heavy moisturizers can blur the pigment over time, Retin-A products (Retinols, Retinoids) or any harsh ingredients especially found in acne medication will prematurely fade the pigment and possible discoloration, same goes with brighteners like Vit-C, Azelaic acid or Kojik acid. Ask them about the kind of cleanser they use and tell them to avoid exfoliating scrubs or cleansers.

All you can do is to advise them on how to go on with their life, caring for their beautifully done and semi-permanently applied pigment. In detail, instructions can be found in the Aftercare form. (Chapter 11)

HEALING STAGES

The healing process can vary from person to person, and the experience may differ. It's important to tell your client to be patient and follow the specific aftercare instructions provided by you. Let them know if they experience unusual swelling, redness or signs of infection during the healing stages to contact you or their healthcare professional for guidance. During the healing stages of microblading, your client can expect several distinct phases as their skin and the pigmented area is undergoing the recovery process. These stages can be scary to the client and they might contact you often for you to reassure them that what they are experiencing is "normal", be patient, informative and most importantly, understanding.

Right after the microblading session, your client's eyebrow may appear darker, sharp and more defined, some clients might fall in love with their eyebrows right away and some might be a little worried; explain to them this is normal because the pigment is fresh and hasn't undergone the healing and settling process. In some cases, redness and minor swelling may be present around the brow area but it usually subsides within a day or two at the most.

First 3 days, or until they start scabbing, the color might intensify and appear even darker. Explain to your client this is the oxidized pigment on the surface and it is temporary.

Some people tend to scab while others don't; either way it's technically normal. Scabbing normally start on day 4 and would probably last 2-3 days or a little longer. However, some clients might be slow healers and would not start scabbing until the second week.

Once the scabbing stage is over, the pigment appears significantly lighter and the strokes might completely disappear at this point; the skin is still healing and the pigment has not settled yet. The provided emoji sheet in chapter-11 helps guiding clients through the healing stages perfectly, make sure to always hand them a sheet on the day of their procedure. The true color will gradually reveal itself as their skin is fully healed 7-10 days after they are done with scabbing.

By the end of the fourth week into the sixth week, the eyebrows should have mostly healed and settled. The pigment should have stabilized and the final results will be more apparent.

INITIAL TOUCH-UP APPOINTMENT

Microblading or any PMU procedure is a two-step process, with the initial session being the first step. The primary purpose of the initial touch-up appointment is to fine-tune and perfect the results of the initial microblading procedure, and it is typically scheduled 6-8 weeks after the initial procedure.

Explain to your clients why this appointment so important; skipping this step may result in less-than-optimal results and a shorter lifespan for her microblading. Over the first few weeks following microblading, the pigment may scab and naturally fade, resulting in uneven healing and imperfection. The 6-8 weeks period allows the skin to heal and the pigment to settle, making it easier for you to make precise adjustments. At the end of the day, you and your client desire the same thing, which is to achieve the best and most long-lasting results.

While the initial procedure lays the foundation, the touch up is the opportunity to perfect the brows, so;

1. When your client come in for her touch up appointment, have her go over the healing stages she experienced after the initial procedure, ask her about the steps she took to care for them (aftercare instructions); you will be surprised how some people never pay attention to all that is written and the verbal instructions you delivered. Assess her healed brows and ask her if she is happy with the color choice and/or the shape thus far,

most clients come back asking for darker color, and that's good (easier to add than to remove), right?

2. You may make adjustments to the shape, color and thickness of the brows based on her feedback and your professional judgment.

3. Clients can have varying healing responses and pigment retention to microblading that can affect the outcome of the procedure, as well as other factors:

   - Some individuals may experience more scabbing or flaking, which can result in more pigment loss. Others may heal more consistently. These individual differences are influenced by factors such as skin type, genetics, overall health.

   - Scar tissue can behave differently when it comes to pigment absorption. It may not retain pigment as well as healthy skin, and this can affect color consistency and retention.

   - How well the client follows the recommended aftercare instructions can also influence the healing and final outcome. Those who don't follow the guidelines may experience issues with pigment retention and/or discoloration.

   - The skills and technique of the artist.

   - The quality of pigments used is also very important for best retention and healed results. Invest well in your pigments; it pays off!

4. After assessing the healed result based on her skin type, you may be able to provide her with new and different aftercare

instructions to maximize pigment retention and better healed results.

ANNUAL TOUCH-UP

The primary purpose of an annual touch up is to maintain the appearance and longevity of microbladed eyebrows. Over time, the pigment naturally fades due to various factors, including sun exposure, skincare products, hormonal fluctuation, and the body's natural metabolizing process. The annual touch up helps refresh and enhance the color and shape of the brows and although it is recommended, it is not always needed as some people can retain and maintain beautiful mircobladed brows longer than a year before needing a touch up. If your client's microblading is not faded enough for the annual touch up, have her wait a bit longer because if you pile up new pigment over halfway faded pigment, it will eventually lead to a solid look, defeating the purpose of microblading natural looks.

Before the annual touch up, it's a good idea to have a mini consultation with your client. This allows you to discuss any changes your client might want, thicker or darker color. You can also go over the aftercare protocol especially if you see evidence in her negligence to caring for her brows.

Skin changes over time and may undergo natural changes that affect how it holds pigment, same goes for health issues that could arise within a period of a year; therefore, it is important to have her fill in a new health history form so you are informed of any new changes to her health.

PERFORMING THE TOUCH-UP

Touch up procedure steps are pretty much the same as the initial procedure except for a few different guidelines strictly regarding stroke application, but in general, you need to do;

- Mini consultation.

- Take photos to document the faded results.

- Discuss and choose the new pigment color with your client if she wishes to go darker.

- During the session, the goal is to refresh and enhance the appearance of the eyebrows, so pay close attention to where the pigment has significantly faded. Only apply strokes in areas where it is needed to maintain symmetry and fill in any gaps. Do not go over areas that are already saturated, as this can lead to over saturation and potentially compromise the final results.

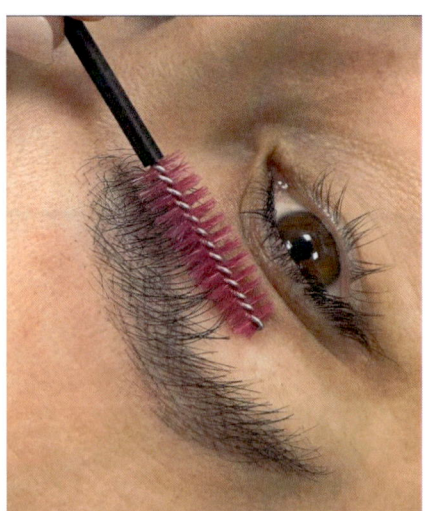

Chapter 16

LICENSING, REGULATIONS

LICENSING

Licensing requirements for permanent makeup artists in the United States can vary significantly from state to state, as each state has its own regulations and licensing procedures. Some states regulate permanent makeup statewide, and others leave it up to counties and cities. To find out the specific licensing requirements in your state, you should contact the appropriate regulatory authority, which is often the state's cosmetology board or Health Department. Here are some common requirements:

- Permanent makeup is classified as a form of tattooing and require artist in some states to obtain a tattoo artist license. This may also involve completing a specific training program and meeting other requirements. Contact your state's health department or relevant licensing agency for information.

- In many states, permanent makeup artists are required to obtain a cosmetology or esthetician license. This typically involves completing a state approved training program and passing an examination. Check with your state's cosmetology board for details.

- You will likely need a general business license to operate your permanent makeup business. Check with your city or county government for the necessary licenses and permits.

- It is crucial to have liability insurance to protect your business and yourself in case of legal claims or adverse reactions.

Regardless of the specific license required, most importantly the individual must obtain the proper training requirement before practicing permanent makeup; enrolling in a reputable training program that meets your state's standard is important. Training must include instructions on health and safety regulation, including infection control and sanitation practices, proper technique and all aspects of the application.

Please remember that regulations and licensing requirements can change over time, so it's crucial to verify the current requirements in your specific state and locality often. Contact the appropriate state agency or board responsible for licensing and regulation in your area to get the most up to date information and guidance. Additionally, joining a professional association for permanent makeup artists like SPCP or the American Academy of Micropigmentation can be a valuable resource for staying informed about the industry standards and licensing requirements in your state.

PRIVACY AND CONFIDENTIALITY

Obtaining a written consent form client before collecting any personal information is important; also, you need to make sure to implement appropriate measures to protect the information you collect, including contact information, medical history, and photographs.

You cannot share any client information or photos without their consent, this applies to sharing information with third parties like social media for marketing purposes.

Safely dispose of any client information that is no longer needed in a manner that protects their privacy (photos, contact information, and health history)

Do not approach clients in public settings; many clients value their beauty secrets privacy.

It's important to note that state and local regulations may also come into play sometimes, and they can vary widely. Some states or local jurisdictions may have additional privacy or data protection laws that govern how permanent makeup provides should handle client information. Although permanent makeup is considered cosmetic, collecting private information especially medical history is important for the procedure. So, maintaining client confidentiality and data protection is important for any professional in the permanent makeup industry.

LIABILITY INSURANCE

Liability insurance, specifically professional liability insurance is very crucial for a permanent makeup business just as it is for many other types of businesses. It helps to protect you and your business in the event of legal claims or lawsuits related to your services.

If a client experiences an adverse reaction, dissatisfaction with the results, or any harm resulting from the procedure, they may file a lawsuit. Liability insurance can help protect your personal assets from being at risk by covering the legal expenses, including attorney's fees and court costs, otherwise you may be personally responsible for covering these costs which can be financially devastating.

It also can enhance your professional credibility and give clients confidence in your services. It shows that you take your business and client safety and satisfaction seriously. Clients may be more likely to choose a permanent makeup artist who is insured because they know there is a safety net in case of any unexpected issues.

Knowing you have liability insurance can provide peace of mind, allowing you to focus on your work without constantly worrying about potential legal challenges, knowing that your business can also continue to operate while dealing with the legal process in the event of any legal claims.

When selecting liability insurance for your permanent makeup business, it's important to consider the specific coverage you need. Be sure to discuss your needs with an insurance agent or broker who can help you tailor a policy to your business. Key components to look for in your policy can include:

- Professional liability: This covers claims related to errors in your services.

- General liability: This covers claims related to accidents, injuries, or property damage on your business premises.

- Product liability: If you sell products related to permanent makeup, this can cover claims related to those products.

- Coverage limits: Ensure your coverage limits are enough to protect your business properly.

Note: Remember to review your insurance policy carefully, understand its terms, and keep it up to date as your business grows or changes. Liability insurance is a smart investment to protect your business and your client's well-being.

Chapter 17

HOW TO GROW YOUR MICROPIGMENTATION BUISNESS

&

HOW TO GROW YOUR BUSINESS ON SOCIAL MEDIA

GROWING YOUR BUSINESS

Growing a permanent makeup business requires a well thought out strategy that combines marketing, customer service, financial planning and effective business management. Define your niche by identifying your target audience and specialization within permanent makeup; this could include microblading, eyeliner, lip blush or scar camouflage. Focusing on a niche can help you stand out and attract clients seeking specific services.

Build a strong online presence, create a professional and user-friendly website that showcases your portfolio, services, pricing, and contact information. Social media is huge and must have, use a platform like Instagram, Facebook, and Pinterest to display your work, share informative content and engage with your audience. Consistency and high-quality visuals are key. You also need to encourage satisfied clients to leave a positive review on platforms like Google, Yelp and social media, that helps to build trust with potential clients.

Optimize your online presence for local search to ensure your business appears in local search results; this includes claiming your Google My Business listing and using location-specific keywords on your website and social media ads.

You need to network with other beauty professionals and local businesses to create mutually beneficial partnerships. For example, collaborating with a spa or salon can lead to client referrals. Also, try to attend beauty industry events, workshops, and conferences to stay informed about trends and to build your professional network.

One of the most essential strategies to build your business is with an excellent reputation by providing excellent customer service and honest communication. Be sincere to their wellbeing and ethical. Word of a mouth is by far the strongest marketing tool you can find.

Develop a comprehensive marketing plan that includes both online and offline strategies. This can involve pay-per-click advertising, email marketing, and content marketing. Use before and after photos to showcase your work and demonstrate the transformation you provide to your clients. You definitely need to leverage the power of social media advertising to target your ideal audience.

Maintain a consistent brand image, including a professional logo, color scheme, and contents that reflects your business's values and personality.

Ensure your pricing is competitive yet reflective of your skills and experience; also, by offering a special promotion or package deals you can attract new clients. Careful not to overdo it, it can signal desperation. Mother's Day, Black Fridays, and other holidays promotes a legit reason to offer special promotions.

Implement a loyalty program to reward repeat clients with discounts or incentives for referring a new customer. For example, I offer my client $25 credit per referral towards their yearly touch ups.

Plan your schedule effectively and manage your time efficiently. Unless you hire people to help you, you might need to balance your time between working on your work schedule, attending to your clients' questions and concerns, social media and marketing, bookkeeping, supplies and inventory. Trust me, you will have your hands full!

Let your clients know that you offer online booking by mentioning it on your website, social media profiles, email signatures and business cards; implementing online booking for your business can streamline appointment management, increase convenience for clients, and improve your overall business operations. There are many platforms to choose from; you just need to find what suits your business in the best way, but in general, you would need an online booking platform that offers payment processing to either pay the full payment of the procedure or booking deposit fee (this can help reduce NO-SHOWS). Also, set up automated confirmation and reminder messages that are sent to clients via email or SMS; this helps reduce the likelihood of missed appointments and of course, one less thing to worry about.

THE IMPORTANCE OF SOCIAL MEDIA TO YOUR BUSINESS

Social media has had a profound impact on communication, information spreading, marketing, and social interaction. It has become a central part of modern life, influencing the way people connect, share, and engage with content and each other. Some of the most well-known social media platforms include Facebook, Instagram, Twitter, LinkedIn, TikTok, YouTube, Pinterest and Snapchat. Each platform has its own unique features and user base, catering to different types of content and communication.

Growing your permanent makeup business on social media is important for several compelling reasons. As we know, social media platforms have billions of active users, providing an enormous potential audience for your business; by establishing a presence on platforms like Instagram, Facebook, and TikTok, you can reach a wide and diverse audience, including potential clients who may not have found you through traditional marketing methods.

It is a powerful tool for building and promoting your brand; consistent and engaging content helps create brand recognition and reinforces your business identity. Your brand identity should reflect the values and qualities that make your permanent makeup business unique. You will be able to engage directly with potential clients by responding to inquiries, providing information or to address any concerns in real time, creating a sense of accessibility and reliability than can enhance client trust.

One of the most important benefits in my opinion, is the ability to showcase your work and talent, visual platforms like Instagram and Pinterest are excellent for showcasing your portfolio. High-quality images and videos of your work can demonstrate your skills and style, attracting clients who appreciate your artistry. It is also an excellent way to educate your audience about permanent makeup and other relevant topics. This helps you to establish an authority in the field and builds trust in your knowledge.

Social media is great to promote special offers, discounts, and promotions to attract new clients and followers that can be potential clients. It is a cost-effective advertising and highly targeted. You can reach specific demographics, interests, and geographic areas with your ads.

Remember that maintaining a consistent and engaging presence on social media requires time and effort. It is essential to develop a content strategy, engage with your audience regularly, and stay up to date with social media trends and best practices. Over time, a well-executed social media strategy can lead to business growth, increased revenue, and an enhanced reputation in the permanent makeup industry. Many of your competitors are likely already active on social media, so establishing a strong presence can give you a competitive advantage in the market.

Remember that business growth takes time, so be patient and persistent in your efforts. Regularly evaluate your strategy and adjust it as needed based on the results you see. Building a strong reputation, providing high-quality work, and maintaining excellent customer service are key elements in the long-term success of your permanent makeup business.

As you close the chapter on your journey to discover the art and science of permanent makeup, I hope you carry with you not only the knowledge and skills you've gained but also the passion and dedication that brought you here.

May your every stroke be filled with creativity and precision, and may your work always bring joy and confidence to those you touch. As you embark on your career, remember that every face is a canvas, every client a unique story waiting to be told.

In this ever-evolving world of beauty, may your artistry continue to flourish, your client relationships deepen, and your business thrive. Keep learning, keep growing, and always pursue excellence.

With warmest regards and the very best wishes for your future in the world of permanent makeup.

God Bless

Printed by Libri Plureos GmbH in Hamburg,
Germany